AF514456

Vocal Fold Injection

대한후두음성언어의학회

The Korean Society of Laryngology, Phoniatrics and Logopedics

Byung-Joo Lee
Tack-Kyun Kwon
Clark A. Rosen
Editors

Vocal Fold Injection

Springer

Editors
Byung-Joo Lee
Department of Otorhinolaryngology
Pusan National University Hospital
Pusan, Korea (Republic of)

Tack-Kyun Kwon
Department of Otorhinolaryngology
College of Medicine, Seoul National University
Seoul, South Korea

Clark A. Rosen
Division of Laryngology
Department of Otolaryngology Head and Neck Surgery
UCSF Voice & Swallowing Center, University of California, San Francisco
California, USA

ISBN 978-981-16-3305-8 ISBN 978-981-16-3303-4 (eBook)
https://doi.org/10.1007/978-981-16-3303-4

© Springer Nature Singapore Pte Ltd. 2021
This work is subject to copyright. All rights are reserved by the Publisher, whether the whole or part of the material is concerned, specifically the rights of translation, reprinting, reuse of illustrations, recitation, broadcasting, reproduction on microfilms or in any other physical way, and transmission or information storage and retrieval, electronic adaptation, computer software, or by similar or dissimilar methodology now known or hereafter developed.
The use of general descriptive names, registered names, trademarks, service marks, etc. in this publication does not imply, even in the absence of a specific statement, that such names are exempt from the relevant protective laws and regulations and therefore free for general use.
The publisher, the authors and the editors are safe to assume that the advice and information in this book are believed to be true and accurate at the date of publication. Neither the publisher nor the authors or the editors give a warranty, expressed or implied, with respect to the material contained herein or for any errors or omissions that may have been made. The publisher remains neutral with regard to jurisdictional claims in published maps and institutional affiliations.

This Springer imprint is published by the registered company Springer Nature Singapore Pte Ltd.
The registered company address is: 152 Beach Road, #21-01/04 Gateway East, Singapore 189721, Singapore

Preface

The textbook *Vocal Fold Injection* is a book written over 3 years, beginning in 2019, as part of the compilation project of the Korean Society of Laryngology, Phoniatrics and Logopedics. The Korean Society of Phoniatrics and Logopedics (KSPL) was founded in October 1980 and changed its name to the Korean Society of Laryngology, Phoniatrics and Logopedics (KSLPL) in 2011. The society has grown into Korea's representative laryngology association, which commemorated its 40th anniversary in 2020.

Vocal fold injection is an important technique that laryngologists must acquire and is being actively performed around the world. Many laryngologists in Korea have also produced esteemed research and papers.

This textbook covers the current state of knowledge on vocal fold injection and includes the most up-to-date information gleaned from the experiences of Korean doctors and renowned experts around the world. It also offers information that is useful for both new and experienced laryngologists who desire to improve their expertise. We tried to incorporate as many images and photographs related to procedures as possible in this book, as well as detailed discussions and essential learning points of procedures to assist readers understand.

We would like to express our deepest gratitude to the members of KSLPL who contributed to the writing as well as distinguished professors from all over the world. As the global COVID-19 pandemic began during the writing period, we are grateful to the writers for completing the writing and proofreading process while caring for patients, providing quarantine and vaccine. We also express our heartfelt condolences to the victims of COVID-19.

Finally, we thank the members of the Textbook Compilation Committee for proofreading this textbook.

September, 2021

Pusan, Republic of Korea — Byung-Joo Lee
Seoul, Republic of Korea — Tack-Kyun Kwon
San Francisco, CA, USA — Clark A. Rosen

Contents

Contributors

Thomas L. Carroll Department of Otolaryngology-Head and Neck Surgery, Harvard Medical School, Boston, MA, USA

Division of Otolaryngology, Department of Surgery, Brigham and Women's Hospital, Boston, MA, USA

Seung-Ho Choi Department of Otorhinolaryngology-Head and Neck Surgery, Asan Medical Center, University of Ulsan College of Medicine, Seoul, South Korea

Shigeru Hirano Department of Otolaryngology Head and Neck Surgery, Kyoto Prefectural University of Medicine, Kyoto, Japan

Woo-Jin Jeong Department of Otorhinolaryngology-Head & Neck Surgery, Seoul National University Bundang Hospital, Seoul National University College of Medicine, Seongnam, South Korea

Han Su Kim Department of Otolaryngology Head and Neck Surgery, College of Medicine, Ewha Womans University, Seoul, South Korea

Seong Keun Kwon Department of Otolaryngology Head and Neck Surgery, Seoul National University College of Medicine, Seoul, South Korea

Tack-Kyun Kwon Department of Otorhinolaryngology-Head and Neck Surgery, Seoul National University College of Medicine, Seoul, South Korea

Byung-Joo Lee Department of Otorhinolaryngology, Pusan National University Hospital, Pusan, Republic of Korea

Sang Hyuk Lee Department of Otolaryngology Head and Neck Surgery, Sungkyunkwan University School of Medicine, Seoul, South Korea

Seung-Won Lee Department of Otolaryngology Head and Neck Surgery, Soonchunhyang University College of Medicine, Bucheon, South Korea

Jae-Yol Lim Department of Otorhinolaryngology, Gangnam Severance Hospital, Yonsei University College of Medicine, Seoul, Republic of Korea

Pavan S. Mallur Department of Otolaryngology Head and Neck Surgery, Harvard Medical School, Boston, MA, USA

Alexandra Mechler-Hickson Division of Otolaryngology Head and Neck Surgery, Department of Surgery, University of Wisconsin-Madison, Madison, WI, USA

Sung Joon Park Department of Otorhinolaryngology-Head and Neck Surgery, College of Medicine, The Catholic University of Korea, Seoul, Republic of Korea

Young-Hak Park Department of Otorhinolaryngology-Head and Neck Surgery, College of Medicine, The Catholic University of Korea, Seoul, Republic of Korea

Clark A. Rosen Division of Laryngology, Department of Otolaryngology Head and Neck Surgery, UCSF Voice & Swallowing Center, University of California, San Francisco, CA, USA

Jin Ho Sohn Department of Otolaryngology-Head and Neck Surgery, Kyungpook National University Chilgok Hospital, Daegu, South Korea

Young-Ik Son Department of Otorhinolaryngology - Head and Neck Surgery, Samsung Medical Center, Sungkyunkwan University School of Medicine, Seoul, South Korea

Susan L. Thibeault Division of Otolaryngology Head and Neck Surgery, Department of Surgery, University of Wisconsin-Madison, Madison, WI, USA

Chen-Chi Wang Department of Otorhinolaryngology-Head & Neck Surgery, Taichung Veterans General Hospital, Taichung, Taiwan

School of Medicine, National Yang Ming Chiao Tung University, Taipei, Taiwan

Department of Audiology and Speech-Language Pathology, Asia University, Taichung, Taiwan

Chi-Te Wang Department of Otolaryngology Head and Neck Surgery, Far Eastern Memorial Hospital, Taipei, Taiwan

Joo Hyun Woo Department of Otorhinolaryngology-Head and Neck Surgery, College of Medicine, Gachon University, Incheon, South Korea

Textbook Compilation Committee

Chair: Tack-Kyun Kwon
Secretary: Doh Young Lee
Members: Han SuKim
Sang Hyuk Lee
Seung-Won Lee
Jae-Yol LIm
Woo-Jin Jeong

Part I

General Considerations and Preoperative Preparations

1 History of Vocal Fold Injection

Sung Joon Park and Young-Hak Park

Abstract

The goal of vocal fold injection is to implant substance at vocal fold and restore characteristics of vocal fold oscillation without adverse reaction. After first description of vocal fold injection in 1911 by Bruening, the evolution of vocal fold injection began with a goal of filling space to achieve glottis competence with an inert material. Recent advances in injection materials and endoscopic technology have broadened the indications of vocal fold injection. Nevertheless, the current challenge is to provide a substance to maintain the space-filling without prohibiting the biomechanical and viscoelastic properties of lamina propria. Because the advances in vocal fold injection have risen from novel materials rather than new technology, the history of vocal fold injection will refer to development of materials.

Keywords

History · Injection laryngoplasty · Injection materials · Cartilage · Bone dust · Tantalum Teflon · Silicone · Gelfoam · Collagen

S. J. Park · Y.-H. Park (✉)
Department of Otorhinolaryngology-Head and Neck Surgery, College of Medicine, The Catholic University of Korea, Seoul, Republic of Korea
e-mail: yhpark7@catholic.ac.kr

1.1 Historical Perspective of Vocal Fold Injection

Injection laryngoplasty, along with medialization thyroplasty and reinnervation surgery, has been considered as the treatment of choice for glottic insufficiency of various etiologies. Among these treatment modalities, injection laryngoplasty has gained its popularity due to its less invasive nature compared to medialization thyroplasty or reinnervation surgery which requires open approach, and its potency to be conducted under in-office settings which enables better anticipation of voice improvement after the treatment. The history of the vocal fold injection is closely related to the development of potential injection materials that can be used. Thus, in this chapter, the authors sought to review the history of the vocal fold injection according to the chronicle of the injection materials that had been used.

1.2 Paraffin

The history of vocal fold injection begins by a German physician named Bruening. In 1911, Bruening reported the first injection laryngoplasty by injecting melted paraffin into the paraglottic space to medialize unilaterally immobile vocal fold for the purpose of treating glottic insufficiency [1]. To perform injection laryngoplasty, Bruening invented a syringe with long 19-gauge needle which enabled injection of

© Springer Nature Singapore Pte Ltd. 2021

B.-J. Lee et al. (eds.), *Vocal Fold Injection*, https://doi.org/10.1007/978-981-16-3303-4_1

paraffin into the immobile vocal fold. This instrument is now called Bruening syringe, which is still used by many physicians to perform injection laryngoplasty. Even though this monumental report has opened the current concept of injection laryngoplasty to overcome the glottic insufficiency by various etiologies, paraffin injection soon became obsolete. The reason for this disuse was due to the *in vivo* characteristics of the paraffin itself. Paraffin caused chronic foreign body reactions with the formation of granuloma, which is later called as paraffinoma [2, 3]. Moreover, extrusion of injected material due to chronic inflammation was observed and when injected in other parts of the body, it failed to retain its place and migrated to unwanted places within human body [2, 3]. As a result, the practice of injection laryngoplasty was largely abandoned shortly after its introduction.

1.3 Cartilage and Bone Paste

1.3.1 Cartilage

Although paraffin injection was abandoned due the side effects of the material itself, the technique of injection laryngoplasty using Bruening syringe had proved its advantages in treatment of glottic insufficiency due to unilateral vocal fold paralysis. As a result, history of search for a new and desirable injectable substance began. Under the assumption that the autologous or homologous materials would produce less tissue reaction than other foreign materials and be less likely to migrate or extrude, Godfrey Edward Arnold revisited injection laryngoplasty and suggested the use of cartilage particles as an injection material [4]. In 1955, Arnold [4] reported functional and histological results of the use of grounded cartilage particles mixed with procaine penicillin G in sesame oil gelatin served as a vehicle in dogs and rabbits, and reported successful outcome. Later on, Arnold [5] mentioned unorganized; rather preliminary results of injecting finely grounded autogenous nasal septal cartilage suspended in gelatin in human subjects in 1957. All cases of laryngeal hemiparalysis or cordectomy treated in this manner were reported to show favorable outcomes with no complications and improved subjective and objective voice.

1.3.2 Bone Paste

In 1960, Goff [6] reported preliminary results of injecting a paste consisting of heterogenous, bovine bone dust suspended in gelatin vehicle for the treatment of laryngeal adductor paralysis. Even though the patients included in this study retained the vocal improvement over several years, issues of allergic reaction to injecting biological substances from different species remained controversial. Hence, no further study results were reported afterwards.

1.3.3 Shortcomings of Cartilage and Bone Paste

Even though the use of autologous cartilage and heterogenous bone paste had shown its value in a good number of cases, it was still not a satisfying injection material for many laryngologists due to various reasons. Cartilage, for instance, must be excised from another part, such as nasal septum, auricle, or rib cartilage, and then prepared by a very meticulous and cumbersome process to ensure the viability of cartilage particles [2–4, 7]. The procedure required a lot of additional work and slightest neglect may lead to the failure of the entire procedure. Moreover, because the injection materials were not entirely inert, the initial vocal improvement were not maintained during the follow up of the patients due to the resorption of the injected material [2, 7]. These shortcomings led to the need for discovery of more improved injection material.

1.4 Tantalum

Tantalum is a rare, very hard, blue-gray, easily fabricated metal with atomic number 73. It is highly conductive of heat and electricity and highly corrosion-resistant. Additionally, favorable reports on minimal tissue reactions to tantalum substances [8] have encouraged researchers to try the powdered metal suspended in glycerin form for use in the injection laryngoplasty. In 1961, Arnold [7] conducted an experiment injecting a suspension of pure tantalum powder in glycerin into the leg muscle of a rabbit and reported that histologic study after 9 months demonstrated an excellent tissue tolerance with very mild foreign body reaction and can easily be handled with the Bruening syringe. Moreover, tantalum oxide was reported to be easily mixed with water or glycerin, and could be readily injected. However, Arnold [7] pointed out that certain technical details of manipulating pure tantalum power through a suitable syringe and needle remained to be a problem. Additionally, it was reported to cause fever for 1 or 2 days after the injection, and the patients felt acutely ill for this period [9]. Due to these clinical drawbacks, only preliminary reports [9] or experimental study results [7] have been reported on the use of tantalum.

1.5 Teflon

1.5.1 Introduction of Teflon

In 1962, Arnold [10] first reported development of Teflon powder mixed with glycerin as an injectable Teflon paste for the use in injection laryngoplasty. In this report, Arnold suggested that Teflon paste appeared to be most suitable for vocal fold injection because it can be well tolerated by the tissue, it is not resorbed by human, and it can be finely dispersed in a harmless vehicle in order to be injectable through the long needle of the Bruening syringe. Teflon is a polymer of tetrafluoroethylene with most inert chemical properties of all known plastic materials then. Microscopic examination results presented in this report showed amorphous foreign body particles surrounded and separated by macrophages in various stages of transformation to fibroblasts, suggesting a process of developing fibrosis. Additionally, giant cells enclosed single particles with a sharp demarcation between this implant and the surrounding muscle into which it appeared to have been injected, and no definite capsule formation had been detected in the younger implant. As a result, Arnold advocated that Teflon paste injection to the paraglottic space, lateral to vocalis muscle, is a safe, effective, and most practical option to treat glottic insufficiency caused by unilateral vocal fold paralysis, congenital dysplastic dysphonia, cordectomy or hemilaryngectomy, and vocal fold defects caused by excessive excision of benign vocal fold lesions. Subsequent reports supported the use of Teflon paste as ideal material for injection laryngoplasty [9, 11–33], and it was eventually approved as an implantable substance by the U.S. Food and Drug Administration (US FDA) in 1972.

1.5.2 Clinical Efficacy and Technical Improvement of Teflon Injection

Numerous case series had been published on the clinical results of Teflon injection laryngoplasty. In 1963, Lewy [9] reported a case with Teflon injection to a patient with UVFP caused by thoracic surgery and concluded that the use of Teflon–glycerin mixture is equally effective but easier to prepare and use compared to tantalum mixture. Subsequent article reported by Arnold in 1963[11] and in 1964[12] concluded that Teflon powder mixed with glycerin is considered as the best substance for injection laryngoplasty on vocal rehabilitation of hemiparalysis and post-cordectomy dysphonia. Rubin [13] reported treatment outcomes of nonreactive synthetics injection for vocal rehabilitation of unilateral vocal fold paralysis, and concluded that silicone absorbed slowly from the injection site and was not enduring while Teflon stayed at the injection site and the improvement was sustained. Von Leden et al. [14] reported consistent improvement of laryngeal function along with aerodynamic, acoustic, and photographic improvements following the injection of Teflon paste into the paralyzed vocal fold.

The technique of Teflon injection improved over the years. In 1973, Dedo et al. [15] reported successful results with of intracordal Teflon injection via indirect laryngoscopy under topical anesthesia for the treatment of 135 patients with dysphonia. In 1975, Carden et al. [16] reported a new method of Teflon injection under general anesthesia by applying thin jet ventilation tube with cuff, positioned at posterior commissure. Furthermore, Ward et al. [17] utilized the flexible and/or rigid fiberoptic systems and popularized a new technique which is still commonly used for injecting various materials into the vocal fold, the transcutaneous transcricothyroid membrane approach. As it will be covered in the following chapters, one of the most important advantages that transcutaneous technique provides, is that it can be done in an in-office setting without sedation and permits more accurate assessment of vocal quality during the procedure [18]. The treatment results of this transcutaneous approach have been dealt by other researchers in many subsequent reports [19–22]. Based on these efforts for improvement, Teflon became the material of choice for injection laryngoplasty until the late 1980s [23].

1.5.3 Tissue Response to Injected Teflon

The response of the laryngeal tissues to which Teflon was injected has also been described. In earlier studies [9, 10] reported within a decade of the introduction of Teflon in injection laryngoplasty, all researchers agreed that a minimum reaction was present and these tissue reactions were always manageable. Subjective response included a moderate degree of local discomfort, and objective response included fairly marked temporary local edema, which required tracheostomy in some cases but eventually subsided with successful end results [9, 10]. Histopathological studies conducted on canine larynx showed that Teflon was inert from a chemical standpoint, with layers of fibrosis observed to be surrounding the implant even after 1.5 years. They observed an absence of migration or extrusion while the squamous epithelium covering the surface of the vocal ligaments remained unchanged, and found no evidence of the carcinogenic effects [24, 25].

Lewy [26] conducted the first histologic evaluation on the response to Teflon from a postmortem specimen of a white male who had received Teflon injection laryngoplasty 17 months prior to his death. This report suggested that Teflon induces inflammatory reaction and fibrosis of the injected tissue which eventually point toward complete fibrosis with disappearance of inflammatory cells, resulting in healing. Moreover, the injected Teflon was inert in appearance with no definite evidence of carcinogenic effects. Subsequent histologic studies substantiated these findings and concluded that Teflon was safe to use in injection laryngoplasty [27–31]. In summary of these reports, the first reaction of larynx to Teflon injection was acute inflammation which involves polymorphonuclear leukocytes and edema around the Teflon. The polymorphonuclear cells are replaced by mononuclear cells, histiocytes, and giant cells within 4–5 days, and only the foreign body granuloma and capsule formation is left without further tissue changes after 3–4 weeks [32].

These histologic responses to Teflon injection also affected the airflow in patients who underwent injection laryngoplasty. Comier et al. [33] reported results on maximum expiratory and inspiratory flow changes prior to and two or more weeks after vocal fold injection with Teflon. They concluded that Teflon injection did not cause a significant reduction in forced expiratory flows and improved inspiratory flows in subjects without evident underlying bronchial disease. Moreover, subsequent reports by Comier et al. [34] concluded that Teflon injection laryngoplasty for unilateral vocal fold paralysis patients created a significant inspiratory airway obstruction within 24 h after injection but it was relieved after 10 days. These results coincide with the timeline of the histologic changes after Teflon injection.

1.5.4 Complications of Teflon

The improper injection of Teflon results not only in less than optimal outcomes, but also in actual worsening of the voice. The laryngeal edema, which develops within 24 h of the Teflon injection due to acute inflammatory reaction described above [34], is one of the unavoidable reactions after Teflon injection laryngoplasty. These laryngeal swelling could cause local swelling, dysphagia, and mild stridor. Tracheostomy might be needed in some of the extreme cases of upper airway obstruction caused by this laryngeal edema [12].

Rubin categorized four technical errors of improper injection of Teflon [35, 36]. First of all, even though Teflon is correctly injected into the most lateral aspect of the thyroarytenoid muscle, overinjection of Teflon produces a convexity of the injected vocal fold surface which, in return induces too much tension at the vibratory surface of vocal fold mucosa, resulting in decreased vibration. Secondly, when Teflon is injected too close to the vocal margin or too medially into the thyroarytenoid muscle, it will not only cause convexity of the cord but also stiffening of the vibratory portion of the vocal fold mucosa resulting hoarseness or diplophonia. This medial injection of Teflon is considered to be the worst technical error for voice improvement, and it causes severe worsening of the voice. The third technical error is Teflon being injected too deeply due to denervation atrophy of the thyroarytenoid muscle, which can cause subglottic deposition of the injected Teflon. This deeply injected Teflon has potential to migrate through cricothyroid space and extralaryngeally into the soft tissue of the neck, causing Teflon granuloma. The last technical error is superficial injection into and beneath the mucus membrane of upper surface of the vocal fold. This error is the least serious of the four, encompassing least potential to affect post-injection voice outcome. In addition to these complications from inadequate injection, Teflon granuloma, teflonoma, was reported to present as a false positive finding in positron emission tomography (PET) of a previously treated thyroid cancer patient [37], false positive in PET-CT of a patient with non-small cell lung cancer [38] and a patient with a history of nasopharyngeal cancer [39], or misdiagnosed as laryngeal cancer in PET-CT [40].

The surgical removal was recommended as the treatment of choice for the improperly injected Teflon. The overinjection or medial injection of Teflon causes convexity of the injected vocal fold surface and needs to be removed [41]. However, in these cases, the injected Teflon forms granuloma or seroma within the thyroarytenoid muscle or Reinkes space, making the removal of injected Teflon without destroying the normal vocal fold tissues almost impossible, rendering it unlikely that the voice can be returned to its pre-injection state [35, 36, 41]. Horn and Dedo [41] reported successful outcomes of case series with 12 patients in which the corrective surgery for overinjection or medial injection of Teflon. The surgical procedures were conducted utilizing mucosal incision at the lateral edge of true vocal fold and removal of injected Teflon only until the vibratory margin of the vocal fold was flattened. Additionally, complete surgical removal was considered as the treatment of choice for teflonomas of the larynx [42, 43], tracheal wall [44], or neck [42] caused by superficially or deeply injected Teflon. For teflonomas of the larynx, various form of lasers had been tested for use in mucosal incision or direct ablation of the teflonomas to minimize the damage to normal larynx [46].

All of the technical errors discussed in the previous paragraphs eventually resulted in the formation of a Teflon granuloma. Classically, formation of granuloma by Teflon injection was initially considered as the process toward healing [24–32]. However, these Teflon granulomas had shown to cause many undesirable symptoms such as dysphonia, airway obstruction, dysphagia, odynophagia, and globus sensation [35, 36, 41]. Additionally, injected Teflon had shown local spread, migration into regional lymphatics, and migration into Reinkes space, causing vocal fold stiffening [45]. These undesirable qualities of Teflon used in injection laryngoplasty led Flint et al. [46] to conclude in 1997 that Teflon is the least desirable among the materials available for vocal fold augmentation. These complications caused one of the most famous material used in injection laryngoplasty since 1962, Teflon, to be abandoned.

1.6 Silicone

1.6.1 Introduction of Silicone

Silicones are synthetic polymers based on the chemical combination of silicon, oxygen, and organic groups. It is a biocompatible material ranging from liquid to solid products and has many applications in medicine. When in fluid form, silicones have a wide range of viscosity depending upon the length of the molecular chain. The certain extent of viscosity provides desirable properties, such as resistance to temperatures required for autoclaving, absence of decomposition or other chemical changes with time, and inertness when implanted in the body, making silicones suitable for medical use. These unique properties of silicones enable it to be easily applied without the need of further preparation process, well tolerated during the sterilization procedure, and injectable using commercially available syringes. This is why the use of silicones in injection laryngoplasty seemed promising [47]. However, while Teflon was considered as a permanent material for injection laryngoplasty, the longevity of liquid Silicone was not as persistent as Teflon. In a preliminary report comparing liquid Silicone and Teflon, Rubin [13] mentioned that liquid Silicone was slowly absorbed from the sites of injection over the course of several months. The viscosity of liquid Silicone was increased in an effort to delay or halt dissipation. However, Silicone in any viscosity showed insignificant amount of remaining injectate within the vocal fold only after 1–4 months. Thus, Rubin advocated the use of liquid Silicone as a temporary material in cases of injection laryngoplasty for unilateral vocal fold paralysis patients with uncertainty of recovery for the purpose of delaying and pre-examining the anticipated effects of the permanent material, Teflon [13, 47].

Even though Silicone had been reported as a temporary injection material for vocal fold augmentation, the US FDA did not authorize its use in injection laryngoplasty. Due to this reason, Silicone was primarily used as injection material in Japan [48]. In contrary to previous report by Rubin, Tsuzuki et al. [48] conducted a histopathologic study of the larynx of a patient who underwent injection laryngoplasty with Silicone solid implant 12 years ago and reported that particles of silicones were encapsulated by thin fibrous tissue within the muscle of the injected vocal fold with no apparent migration beyond the adjacent vocalis. Only a few foreign body giant cells and minimal cellular infiltration were present with no definite evidence of dysplasia nor metaplasia and no carcinogenic effect was observed. Moreover, according to the survey results from 54 patients who underwent injection laryngoplasty 3–16 years prior to the survey, no evident laryngeal disease was induced by Silicone solid implant injection laryngoplasty [48]. In addition to this report, several other studies demonstrated minimal immediate foreign body reaction or inflammatory reaction to Silicone when injected into the vocal folds of experimental animals and humans [47, 49, 50]. Moreover, Tsuzuki et al. [51] reported that both liquid and solid implant of Silicone for injection laryngoplasty were effective in improving the voices for 33 patients with unilateral vocal fold paralysis. They further categorized Silicone implant, and suggested that liquid Silicone was useful for temporary voice improvement due to its ultimate absorption while solid Silicone was not absorbed and is therefore as effective as Teflon in the long-term follow up. These findings supported the use of Silicone in liquid or solid implant form to be used in injection laryngoplasty.

1.6.2 Development of Improved Form of Silicone

To improve the ease and efficacy of injection while improving the longevity of the material, modification of Silicone injection material was conducted. As a result, polydimethylsiloxane (PDMS, Bioplastique™ until 2001, Vox Implants™ after 2001), which consisted of a 60/40 mixture of textured solid silicone elastomer particles with a mean particle diameter of 200um suspended in bioexcretable gel (low molecular weight polyvinylpyrrlidone hydrogel) and injectable with a 27-gauze needle was introduced [52–60]. The PDMS was utilized in the medical field in 1989, mainly in plastic surgery [61] or urology [62, 63]. The use of PDMS as injection material was first mentioned in the European literature by Hofler and Duman, in 1993 [52]. The PDMS did not induce uncontrollable, acute, or chronic inflammatory reactions involving the formation of giant cell granulomas and did not migrate or was absorbed in the human body, which are advantages of Silicone over Teflon [52–60].

Moreover, long-term studies conducted on PDMS showed similar persistency which were achieved in Teflon [52–60]. Therefore, PDMS was once considered as an ideal permanent alternatives of Teflon, for injection laryngoplasty.

1.6.3 Shortcoming of Silicone

Even though various forms of Silicone seemed to be adequate alternatives for Teflon, quite a few shortcomings of Silicone used in injection laryngoplasty have been reported in the literature. Fukuda [64] reported a foreign body reaction and a carcinogenic effect shown in one human larynx who had undergone injection laryngoplasty with Silicone solid implant 2 months prior. Kumagai et al. [65] reported occurrence of 18 cases and reviewed 28 additional cases of connective tissue disease following the injection of liquid or solid implant of Silicone for cosmetic purposes. Moreover, Henly et al. [66] reported local and distant migration of small silicone particles in animals that received a silicone injection for urinary incontinence. In addition to these shortcomings, Winer et al. [67] first described the granulomatous reactions in soft tissues of patients who received liquid Silicone injections and named it siliconoma. Furthermore, Baijens et al. [68] reported the first rejection response of PDMS resulting in extrusion of the injected material and repeated granulomatous inflammation after injection laryngoplasty. For the treatment of siliconoma, similar to the recommended treatment for Teflonoma, complete surgical excision was recommended in this paper. In 2008, Randhawa et al. [69] reported another case of foreign body reaction and possible migration of PDMS. They concluded that, despite the low possibility, the risk of foreign body reaction and migration is still present for PDMS when used in injection laryngoplasty. In the same year, Echternach et al. [60] reported a case with severe dysphonia accompanied by decreased vibration capacity of the vocal fold after misinjected PDMS, which required partial explantation. Even though the partial removal improved the mucosal waves and increased the amplitudes, only slight improvement of the voice was achieved. Consequently, the authors emphasized that the correct positioning of the PDMS injection is as important as using Teflon for injection laryngoplasty. Therefore, injecting too medially into the vocalis muscle should be avoided in all circumstances when using PDMS for injection laryngoplasty. Similar to that in Teflon, false positive findings on PET-CT images after PDMS injection laryngoplasty for unilateral vocal fold paralysis in a patient with non-small cell lung cancer was also reported [70]. These shortcomings of Silicone and the development of other better materials have eventually caused the use of Silicone for injection laryngoplasty to be considered as an obsolete technique by late 2000s.

1.7 Gelfoam

Gelfoam or SURGIFOAM® is an absorbable gelatin sponge like preparation which was initially developed as a hemostatic material [71]. In foam form, it may act as a scaffold for fibrous tissue ingrowth when soaked with blood [72]. In powder form, it was used as a dressing material for open wounds and as a hemostatic material for bone bleeding [71]. The advantage of gelfoam was that it had excellent tissue tolerance, with gradual absorption potency. Gelfoam was reported to last for 2–5 weeks when it is placed in muscle [73]. The rate of absorption is known to depend upon the density of the implanted material and the metabolic activity of the recipient tissue [71]. Despite this temporary nature, gelfoam was first introduced in laryngology, and was initially used in injection laryngoplasty of temporary purpose for patients with glottis insufficiency due to unilateral vocal fold paralysis and who were contraindications for the use of permanent injection materials, such as Teflon or Silicone, due to its indefinite permanency.

In 1978, Schramm et al. [71] described the preparation method for its use in injection laryngoplasty, and reported the outcome in 25 patients with unilateral vocal fold paralysis. The viscosity of the injected form, which is a mixture of sterile gelfoam powder and normal saline, was nearly same as that of Teflon paste. Hence, Bruening syringe was used for injections. Even though they reported one case of a superficially injected patient who presented extrusion of injected material 2 weeks after, other 24 patients showed only minimal inflammatory reactions afterwards. The first 3 or 4 weeks following the injection showed little changes in the augmented vocal fold, while these bulks gradually decreased over the next 4–6 weeks. Eventually, the volume augmented by gelfoam injection subsided completely by the tenth week after the injection laryngoplasty.

Due to this temporary nature, gelfoam injection laryngoplasty was utilized in cases of temporary vocal fold injection [74–77] or trial injection [71, 78] to anticipate the efficacy of permanent injection. However, the need of inconvenient pre-injection preparation procedure and the demand for discovery of new long-lasting injection material have led to the current abandonment of gelfoam use in injection laryngoplasty.

1.8 Collagen

The concern on acute and/or chronic inflammatory reactions to alloplastic polymers as an injection material motivated researchers to consider the use of homologous or heterologous components of a living organism with acceptable longevity as an alternative injectable substances. In this sense, collagen was an attractive substance because it is a natural constituent of the normal extracellular matrix protein of the deep lamina propria or vocal ligament and fulfills the criteria for a suitable bio-filler. One of the biggest concerns was to sufficiently reduce the antigenicity of collagen without destroying the essential structural components. Enzymatic digestion of the non-helical portions (telopeptides) of the collagen molecule has enabled the solubilization of the collagen, and chemical modification, so called crosslinking, has stabilized the collagen, rendering it suitable to be used as injectable filler material [79].

1.8.1 Exogenous Collagen (Heterologous Bovine Collagen, Zyderm® or Zyplast®)

Historically, collagen from bovine sources was isolated and purified in the middle of the 1970s as a filler material for aesthetic purposes [2]. After several years of clinical investigations done by aesthetic surgeons, injectable collagen implants were approved for medical use by the US FDA in 1981 [79]. The successful and lasting results for the treatment of dermal deficiencies with bovine collagen, brought attention to using bovine collagen preparations in injection laryngoplasty. In 1984, Ford et al. [80] conducted the first use of bovine collagen for vocal fold injection in a canine model. When compared with Teflon, there was significant absence of foreign body reaction with only a few scattered histiocytes and no giant cells. Ingrowth of fibroblast was present, capillary ingrowth was evident, and submucosal injection was reported as feasible. In the following animal experiment, Ford [81] also advocated that collagen should be injected in the plane of the vocal ligament for best results. An injection made too deeply will induce rapid resorption, while an injection into the superficial layer of the lamina propria will stiffen the vocal fold, impairing the normal vocal fold vibration. In 1986, Ford and Bless [82, 83] reported their clinical experience with injectable collagen for vocal fold augmentation and showed that improved glottic efficiency was relatively persistent during the study period with only slight decrement over 1 year. The best improvements were achieved in patients with unilateral vocal fold paralysis, while bilaterally scarred vocal folds did not appear to respond optimally to the treatment. Only one patient was reported to experience a delayed hypersensitivity reaction.

Problems with bovine collagen injection rose primarily from potential allergic reaction to the xenograft proteins. Physicians who were planning to use collagen implants must first question the patient of a personal or family history of connective tissue diseases [84]. In addition, the patient needs to undergo a collagen skin test to screen for pre-existing allergy to the bovine collagen and be monitored for 6 weeks [2, 3]. However, a thorough medical history taking and skin test are not always sufficient to identify patients who will show hypersensitivity to collagen implants [85]. Some authors postulate that hypersensitivity reaction after a negative skin test can occur in as many as 3% of patients [86]. Due to the possibility of life-threatening airway obstruction by allergic reactions caused after vocal fold injection with collagen, the US FDA never approved collagen for intralaryngeal injection. For these reasons, bovine collagen never gained popularity, and there have only been a few reports on its use in injection laryngoplasty [82, 83, 86–88].

1.8.2 Human Collagen

1.8.2.1 Autologous Collagen (Purified Human Forms of Autologous Collagen)

The autologous purified human forms of collagen were then utilized to avoid the unpredictable host-graft reaction by bovine collagen. The researchers hypothesized that collagen extracted from patients' own source would be ideal for use in injection. As a result, recipient served as their own donors by extracting collagen from their own skin. Injection of this autologous collagen revealed its intradermal persistence up to 6 months with minimal inflammatory reaction and ingrowth of native fibroblasts [2, 89]. In 1995, Ford et al. [90] reported the first preliminary clinical study results of autologous collagen used in injection laryngoplasty for patients with non-paralyzed glottic insufficiencies. The results indicated that autologous collagen was comparable to bovine collagen and the likelihood of a hypersensitivity response was negligible. The effect of autologous collagen injection laryngoplasty lasted stable upto 6 months in this paper, and was anticipated to persist longer than bovine collagen due to the unnecessity of additional procedures to eliminate antigenicity. Similar treatment results of autologous collagen injection laryngoplasty lasting upto 6 months were subsequently reported [91, 92]. Despite all these advantages, autologous collagen had limitations to be used in clinical settings, such as the inevitable donor site morbidity, the required delay in implant availability owing to processing time, and the increased cost associated with individual graft preparation. Thus, autologous collagen has not been used widely in injection laryngoplasty.

1.8.2.2 Homologous Collagen (Purified Forms of Human Collagen from Homologous Cadaveric Skin, Micronized Acellular Derma Compound, Cymetra®)

A need for readily available form of homogenous collagen, to overcome the shortcomings of autologous collagen for injection laryngoplasty, brought attention to purified forms of human collagen from cadaveric skin. Cymetra®, a commercially available form of micronized acellular dermal compound produced from cadaveric dermal tissue, was developed. The removal of all cells from cadaveric dermis results in a graft with low immunogenicity and with all of the above-mentioned advantages of using collagen for vocal fold injection [93–95]. Even though Lundy et al. [96] attained results with Cymetra that were comparable to type I thyroplasty, validation of their results was lacking in the further literature. Karpenko et al. [97] found that voice improvements were not maintained over a 3 month period for unilateral vocal cord paralysis. Due to its inconsistent results reported in injection laryngoplasty owing to various degree of absorption afterwards, Cymetra received US FDA approval for skin augmentation but never for injection laryngoplasty (Table 1.1).

Table 1.1 Comparison of materials included in this chapter for injection laryngoplasty

Material	Location of injection	Amount injected	Duration	Viscosity	Needle gauge	US FDA approval for injection laryngoplasty (at any time)
Paraffin	Lateral to vocal ligament	Exact amount	Permanent	Low	18–19	No
Cartilage	Lateral to vocal ligament	Overinject	1–3 months	Low	18–19	No
Bone paste	Lateral to vocal ligament	Overinject	1–3 months	Low	18–19	No
Tantalum	Lateral to vocal ligament	Slightly overinject	Permanent	Low	18–19	No
Teflon	Lateral to vocal ligament	Exact amount	Permanent	Low	18–19	Yes
Silicone	Lateral to vocal ligament	Slightly overinject	3–6 months or permanent	Variable	18–19	No
Gelfoam	Lateral to vocal ligament	Overinject	1–3 months	High	18–22	No
Bovine collagen	Within the vocal ligament	Overinject	6 months	High	27	No
Human collagen	Within the vocal ligament	Overinject	6 months	High	27–30	No
Cymetra	Within the vocal ligament	Overinject	6–9 months	Low	22	No

Key Learning Points:

- The history of injection laryngoplasty began in 1911, but soon it was abandoned for decades.
- The injection laryngoplasty has regained its fame from 1950s when autologous cartilage and heterogenous bone dust was evaluated for use.
- The bio-materials used in the early periods had limitation due to the temporary effects caused by absorption after injection.
- Synthetic polymers suspended in a biocompatible carrier, such as Teflon or Silicone, was commonly used and was once considered as materials of choice, due to its persistence of effect.
- However, acute and/or chronic inflammatory reaction to these foreign materials and the complications associated with migration of these synthetic materials prohibited its use in injection laryngoplasty.
- The development and the use of natural component of normal vocal fold, such as collagen, has been attempted but with limitations regarding the consistent augmenting effects after injection laryngoplasty.
- Further search for ideal material with minimal antigenicity and consistent persistence after injection is still on going for injection laryngoplasty.

References

1. Bruening W. Uber eine neue Behandlungsmethode der Rekurrenslahmung. Verh Dtsch Laryg. 1911;18:23.
2. Courey MS. Injection laryngoplasty. Otolaryngol Clin N Am. 2004;37(1):121–38. https://doi.org/10.1016/j.otc.2003.12.002.
3. O'Leary MA, Grillone GA. Injection laryngoplasty. Otolaryngol Clin N Am. 2006;39(1):43–54. https://doi.org/10.1016/j.otc.2005.10.008.
4. Arnold GE. Vocal rehabilitation of paralytic dysphonia. I. Cartilage injection into a paralyzed vocal cord. AMA Arch Otolaryngol. 1955;62(1):1–17. https://doi.org/10.1001/archotol.1955.03830010003001.
5. Arnold GE. Vocal rehabilitation of paralytic dysphonia. III. Present concepts of laryngeal paralysis. AMA Arch Otolaryngol. 1957;65(4):317–36. https://doi.org/10.1001/archotol.1957.03830220001001.
6. Goff WF. Laryngeal adductor paralysis treated by vocal cord injection of bone paste; a preliminary investigation. Trans Pac Coast Otoophthalmol Soc Annu Meet. 1960;41:77–88.
7. Arnold GE. Vocal rehabilitation of paralytic dysphonia. VI. Further studies of intracordal injection materials. Arch Otolaryngol. 1961;73:290–4. https://doi.org/10.1001/archotol.1961.00740020298007.
8. Bailey OT, Ingraham FD, Weadon PS, Susen AF. Tissue reactions to powdered tantalum in the central nervous system. J Neurosurg. 1952;9(1):83–92. https://doi.org/10.3171/jns.1952.9.1.0083.
9. Lewy RB. Glottic reformation with voice rehabilitation in vocal cord paralysis. The injection of Teflon and tantalum. Laryngoscope. 1963;73:547–55. https://doi.org/10.1288/00005537-196305000-00007.
10. Arnold GE. Vocal rehabilitation of paralytic dysphonia: IX. Technique of intracordal injection. Arch Otolaryngol. 1962;76(4):358–68. https://doi.org/10.1001/archotol.1962.00740050368013.
11. Arnold GE. Vocal rehabilitation of paralytic dysphonia: X. functional results of intrachordal injection. Arch Otolaryngol. 1963;78(2):81–8. https://doi.org/10.1001/archotol.78.2.81.
12. Arnold GE. Further experiences with intracordal Teflon injection. Laryngoscope. 1964;74:802–15. https://doi.org/10.1288/00005537-196406000-00004.
13. Rubin HJ. Dysphonia due to unilateral nerve paralysis. Treatment by the intracordal injection of synthetics - a preliminary report. Calif Med. 1965;102(2):105–9.
14. Von Leden H, Yanagihara N, Werner-Kukuk E. Teflon in unilateral vocal cord paralysis. Preoperative and postoperative function studies. Arch Otolaryngol. 1967;85(6):666–74. https://doi.org/10.1001/archotol.1967.00760040668014.
15. Dedo HH, Urrea RD, Lawson L. Intracordal injection of Teflon in the treatment of 135 patients with dysphonia. Ann Otol Rhinol Laryngol. 1973;82(5):661–7. https://doi.org/10.1177/000348947308200509.
16. Carden E, Browder JP, Fischer ND. Teflon injection of vocal cords under general anesthesia: a new method. Anesth Analg. 1975;54(6):739–41. https://doi.org/10.1213/00000539-197511000-00015.
17. Ward PH, Hanson DG, Abemayor E. Transcutaneous Teflon injection of the paralyzed vocal cord: a new technique. Laryngoscope. 1985 Jun;95(6):644–9. https://doi.org/10.1288/00005537-198506000-00002.
18. Ford CN, Roy N, Sandage M, Bless DM. Rigid endoscopy for monitoring indirect vocal fold injection. Laryngoscope. 1998;108(10):1584–6. https://doi.org/10.1097/00005537-199810000-00030.
19. McCaffrey TB, Lipton R. Transcutaneous Teflon injection for paralytic dysphonia. Laryngoscope. 1989;99(5):497–9. https://doi.org/10.1288/00005537-198905000-00006.

20. Strasnick B, Berke GS, Ward PH. Transcutaneous Teflon injection for unilateral vocal cord paralysis: an update. Laryngoscope. 1991;101(7 Pt 1):785–7. https://doi.org/10.1288/00005537-199107000-00017.
21. Feinmesser R, Segal K, Gertel M. Transcutaneous Teflon injection of the paralyzed vocal cord: an improvised technique. J Otolaryngol. 1993;22(3):148–9.
22. McCaffrey TV. Transcutaneous Teflon injection for vocal cord paralysis. Otolaryngol Head Neck Surg. 1993;109(1):54–9. https://doi.org/10.1177/019459989310900110.
23. Sadek SAA, Nassar WY, Tobias MA. Teflon injection of the vocal cords under general anesthesia. J Laryngol Otol. 1987;101:695–705.
24. Kirchner FR, Toledo PS, Svoboda DJ. Studies of the larynx after teflon injection. Arch Otolaryngol. 1966;83(4):350–4. https://doi.org/10.1001/archotol.1966.00760020352013.
25. Toomey JM, Brown BS. The histological response to intracordal injection of teflon paste. Laryngoscope. 1967;77(1):110–20. https://doi.org/10.1288/00005537-196701000-00010.
26. Lewy RB. Responses of laryngeal tissue to granular teflon in situ. Arch Otolaryngol. 1966;83(4):355–9. https://doi.org/10.1001/archotol.1966.00760020357014.
27. Stone JW, Arnold GE. Human larynx injected with Teflon paste. Histological study of innervation and tissue reaction. Arch Otolaryngol. 1967;86(5):550–61. https://doi.org/10.1001/archotol.1967.00760050552014.
28. Harris HE Jr, Hawk WA. Laryngeal injection of teflon paste. Report of a case with postmortem study of the larynx. Arch Otolaryngol. 1969;90(2):194–7. https://doi.org/10.1001/archotol.1969.00770030196021.
29. Stone JW, Arnold GE, Stephens CB. Intracordal polytef (Teflon) injection. Histologic study of three further cases. Arch Otolaryngol. 1970;91(6):568–74. https://doi.org/10.1001/archotol.1970.00770040798014.
30. Goff WF. Intracordal polytef (teflon) injection. Histologic study of two cases. Arch Otolaryngol. 1973;97(5):371–2. https://doi.org/10.1001/archotol.1973.00780010383002.
31. Lewy RB. Experience with vocal cord injection. Ann Otol Rhinol Laryngol. 1976;85(4 Pt 1):440–50. https://doi.org/10.1177/000348947608500404.
32. Lewy RB, Millet D. Immediate local tissue reactions to Teflon vocal cord implants. Laryngoscope. 1978;88(8 Pt 1):1339–42. https://doi.org/10.1288/00005537-197808000-00016.
33. Cormier Y, Kashima H, Summer W, Menkes H. Airflow in unilateral vocal cord paralysis before and after Teflon injection. Thorax. 1978;33(1):57–61. https://doi.org/10.1136/thx.33.1.57.
34. Cormier Y, Kashima H, Summer W. Subclinical reduction in airflows after Teflon injection of vocal cord. Laryngoscope. 1980;90(6 Pt 1):1027–31. https://doi.org/10.1002/lary.1980.90.6.1027.
35. Rubin HJ. Pitfalls in treatment of dysphonias by intracordal injection of synthetics. Laryngoscope. 1965;75(9):1381–97. https://doi.org/10.1288/00005537-196509000-00001.
36. Rubin HJ. Misadventures with injectable polytef (Teflon). Arch Otolaryngol. 1975;101(2):114–6. https://doi.org/10.1001/archotol.1975.00780310036010.
37. Yeretsian RA, Blodgett TM, Branstetter BF 4th, Roberts MM, Meltzer CC. Teflon-induced granuloma: a false-positive finding with PET resolved with combined PET and CT. AJNR Am J Neuroradiol. 2003;24(6):1164–6.
38. Truong MT, Erasmus JJ, Macapinlac HA, Podoloff DA. Teflon injection for vocal cord paralysis: false-positive finding on FDG PET-CT in a patient with non-small cell lung cancer. AJR Am J Roentgenol. 2004;182(6):1587–9. https://doi.org/10.2214/ajr.182.6.1821587.
39. Chadwick JL, Khalid A, Wagner H, Stack BC Jr. Teflon granuloma results in a false-positive "second primary" on 18F-2-deoxyglucose positron emission tomography in a patient with a history of nasopharyngeal cancer. Am J Otolaryngol. 2007;28(4):251–3. https://doi.org/10.1016/j.amjoto.2006.08.016.
40. Ondik MP, Kang J, Bayerl MG, Bruno M, Goldenberg D. Teflon laryngeal granuloma presenting as laryngeal cancer on combined positron emission tomography and computed tomography scanning. J Laryngol Otol. 2009;123(5):575–8. https://doi.org/10.1017/S0022215108003988. Epub 2008 Oct 31
41. Horn KL, Dedo HH. Surgical correction of the convex vocal cord after Teflon injection. Laryngoscope. 1980;90(2):281–6. https://doi.org/10.1288/00005537-198002000-00013.
42. Wenig BM, Heffner DK, Oertel YC, Johnson FB. Teflonomas of the larynx and neck. Hum Pathol. 1990;21(6):617–23. https://doi.org/10.1016/s0046-8177(96)90008-8.
43. Hsiung MW, Lin YL. Lateral thyrotomy with strap muscle transposition for Teflon granuloma. Eur Arch Otorhinolaryngol. 2005;262(4):298–301. https://doi.org/10.1007/s00405-004-0821-1.
44. McCarthy MP, Gideon JK, Schnadig VJ. A teflon granuloma presenting as an endotracheal nodule. Chest. 1993;104(1):311–3. https://doi.org/10.1378/chest.104.1.311.
45. Lano CF Jr, Reinisch L, Ossoff RH, Garrett CG, Kuo T, Bryant GL Jr, et al. Ablation of Teflon granulomas in the canine larynx with the free-electron laser. Ann Otol Rhinol Laryngol. 1999;108(1):17–23. https://doi.org/10.1177/000348949910800103.
46. Flint PW, Corio RL, Cummings CW. Comparison of soft tissue response in rabbits following laryngeal implantation with hydroxylapatite, silicone rubber, and Teflon. Ann Otol Rhinol Laryngol. 1997;106(5):399–407. https://doi.org/10.1177/000348949710600508.
47. Rubin HJ. Intracordal injection of silicone in selected dysphonias. Arch Otolaryngol. 1965 Jun;81:604–7. https://doi.org/10.1001/archotol.1965.00750050619014.
48. Tsuzuki T, Fukuda H, Fujioka T. Response of the human larynx to silicone. Am J

Otolaryngol. 1991;12(5):288–91. https://doi.org/10.1016/0196-0709(91)90007-3.
49. Donnellan WL, Gabriel W, Maurizi DG, Holinger PH. The use of silastic in the treatment of unilateral cord paralysis. An experimental study. Ann Otol Rhinol Laryngol. 1966;75(3):646–56. https://doi.org/10.1177/000348946607500305.
50. Saito S. Phonosurgery-basic study on the mechanism of phonation and endolaryngeal microsurgery. Otol Fukuoka. 1977;23:235–42.
51. Tsuzuki T, Fukuda H, Fujioka T, Takayama E, Kawaida M. Voice prognosis after liquid and solid silicone injection. Am J Otolaryngol. 1991;12(3):165–9. https://doi.org/10.1016/0196-0709(91)90148-9.
52. Hofler H, Duman M. Stimmlippenunterfiitterung mit Bioplastique:erste Ergebnisse. Zentralbl HNO. 1993;577
53. Alves CB, Loughran S, MacGregor FB, Dey JIR, Bowie LJ. Bioplastique medialization therapy improves the quality of life in terminally ill patients with vocal cord palsy. Clin Otolaryngol Allied Sci. 2002;27(5):387–91. https://doi.org/10.1046/j.1365-2273.2002.00601.x.
54. Duruisseau O, Wagner I, Fugain C, Chabolle F. Endoscopic rehabilitation of vocal cord paralysis with a silicone elastomer suspension implant. Otolaryngol Head Neck Surg. 2004;131(3):241–7. https://doi.org/10.1016/j.otohns.2003.11.021.
55. Bernal-Sprekelsen M, Caballero M, Farrè X, Calvo C, Alòs L. Particulate silicone for vocal fold augmentation: morphometric evaluation in a rabbit model. Ann Otol Rhinol Laryngol. 2004;113(3 Pt 1):234–41. https://doi.org/10.1177/000348940411300313.
56. Sittel C, Echternach M, Federspil PA, Plinkert PK. Polydimethylsiloxane particles for permanent injection laryngoplasty. Ann Otol Rhinol Laryngol. 2006;115(2):103–9. https://doi.org/10.1177/000348940611500204.
57. Hamilton DW, Sachidananda R, Carding PN, Wilson JA. Bioplastique injection laryngoplasty: voice performance outcome. J Laryngol Otol. 2007;121(5):472–5. https://doi.org/10.1017/S0022215106005275.
58. Hagemann M, Seifert E. The use of polydimethylsiloxane for injection laryngoplasty. World J Surg. 2008;32(9):1940–7. https://doi.org/10.1007/s00268-008-9619-4.
59. Bergamini G, Alicandri-Ciufelli M, Molteni G, Villari D, Luppi MP, Genovese E, et al. Therapy of unilateral vocal fold paralysis with polydimethylsiloxane injection laryngoplasty: our experience. J Voice. 2010;24(1):119–25. https://doi.org/10.1016/j.jvoice.2008.05.003.
60. Echternach M, Delb W, Wagner M, Sittel C, Verse T, Richter B. Polydimethylsiloxane in the human vocal fold: description of partial explantation. Laryngoscope. 2008;118(2):375–7. https://doi.org/10.1097/MLG.0b013e31815a9eea.
61. Ersek RA, Gregory SR, Salisbury AY. Bioplastique at 6 years: clinical outcome studies. Plast Reconstr Surg. 1997;100(6):1570–4. https://doi.org/10.1097/00006534-199711000-00031.
62. Guys JM, Sirneoni-Alias J, Fakhro A, Delarue A. Use of polydimethylsiloxane for endoscopic treatment of neurogenic urinary incontinence in children. J Urol. 1999;162(6):2133–5. https://doi.org/10.1016/s0022-5347(05)68141-4.
63. Harriss DR, Iacovou LW, Lemberger RL. Periurethral silicone microimplants (Macroplastique) for the treatment of genuine stress incontinence. Br J Urol. 1996;78(5):722–8. https://doi.org/10.1046/j.1464-410x.1996.17510.x.
64. Fukuda H. Silicone injection into vocal fold for vocal rehabilitation. Nippon Jibiinkoka Gakkai Kaiho. 1970;73:92–112.
65. Kumagai Y, Shiokawa Y, Medsger TA Jr, Rodnan GP. Clinical spectrum of connective tissue disease after cosmetic surgery. Observations on eighteen patients and a review of the Japanese literature. Arthritis Rheum. 1984;27(1):1–12. https://doi.org/10.1002/art.1780270101.
66. Henly DR, Barrett DM, Weiland TL, O'Connor MK, Malizia AA, Wein AJ. Particulate silicone for use in periurethral injections: local tissue effects and search for migration. J Urol. 1995;153(6): 2039–43.
67. Winer LH, Sternberg TH, Lehman R, Ashley FL. Tissue reactions to injected silicone liquids. A report of three cases. Arch Dermatol. 1964;90:588–93. https://doi.org/10.1001/archderm.1964.01600060054010.
68. Baijens L, Speyer R, Linssen M, Ceulen R, Manni JJ. Rejection of injectable silicone "Bioplastique" used for vocal fold augmentation. Eur Arch Otorhinolaryngol. 2007;264(5):565–8. https://doi.org/10.1007/s00405-006-0224-6.
69. Randhawa PS, Ramsay AD, Rubin JS. Foreign body reaction to polymethylsiloxane gel (Bioplastique) after vocal fold augmentation. J Laryngol Otol. 2008;122(7):750–3. https://doi.org/10.1017/S002221510800193X.
70. Tessonnier L, Fakhry N, Taieb D, Giovanni A, Mundler O. False-positive finding on FOG-PET/CT after injectable elastomere implant (Vox implant) for vocal cord paralysis. Otolaryngol Head Neck Surg. 2008;139(5):738–9. https://doi.org/10.1016/j.otohns.2008.07.033.
71. Schramm VL, May M, Lavorato AS. Gelfoam paste injection for vocal cord paralysis: temporary rehabilitation of glottic incompetence. Laryngoscope. 1978;88(8 Pt 1):1268–73. https://doi.org/10.1288/00005537-197808000-00007.
72. Joseph RB. The effect of absorbable gelatin sponge preparations and other agents on scar formation in the dog's middle ear. An experimental histopathologic study. Laryngoscope. 1962;72:1528–48. https://doi.org/10.1288/00005537-196211000-00003.
73. Jenkins HP, Clarke JS. Gelatin sponge, a new hemostatic substance; studies on absorbability. Arch Surg. 1945;51:253–61. https://doi.org/10.1001/archsurg.1945.01230040262005.

74. Miller MA, Saltvoll B. Absorbable gelatin powder injection for transient vocal cord paralysis. AORN J. 1995;61(5):821–6. https://doi.org/10.1016/s0001-2092(06)63714-9.
75. Hoffman HT, Sullivan MJ, Winter P. Gelfoam injection for vocal cord paralysis prior to radiation therapy. Ear Nose Throat J. 1991;70(6):385–6.
76. Anderson TD, Mirza N. Immediate percutaneous medialization for acute vocal fold immobility with aspiration. Laryngoscope. 2001;111(8):1318–21. https://doi.org/10.1097/00005537-200108000-00002.
77. Coskun HH, Rosen CA. Gelfoam injection as a treatment for temporary vocal fold paralysis. Ear Nose Throat J. 2003;82(5):352–3.
78. Carroll TL, Rosen CA. Trial vocal fold injection. J Voice. 2010;24(4):494–8. https://doi.org/10.1016/j.jvoice.2008.11.001.
79. Stenzel KH, Miyata T, Rubin AL. Collagen as a biomaterial. Annu Rev Biophys Bioeng 1974;3(0): 231–253. doi:https://doi.org/10.1146/annurev.bb.03.060174.001311.
80. Ford CN, Martin DW, Warner TF. Injectable collagen in laryngeal rehabilitation. Laryngoscope. 1984;94(4):513–8. https://doi.org/10.1288/00005537-198404000-00016.
81. Ford CN. Histological studies on the fate of soluble collagen injected into canine vocal folds. Laryngoscope. 1986;96(11):1248–57. https://doi.org/10.1002/lary.1986.96.11.1248.
82. Ford CN, Bless DM. A preliminary study of injectable collagen in human vocal fold augmentation. Otolaryngol Head Neck Surg. 1986;94(1):104–12. https://doi.org/10.1177/019459988609400117.
83. Ford CN, Bless DM. Clinical experience with injectable collagen for vocal fold augmentation. Laryngoscope. 1986;96(8):863–9. https://doi.org/10.1002/lary.1986.96.8.863.
84. Ford CN, Gilchrist KW, Bartell TE. Persistence of injectable collagen in the human larynx: a histopathologic study. Laryngoscope. 1987;97(6):724–7. https://doi.org/10.1288/00005537-198706000-00015.
85. Hanke CW, Robinson JK. Injectable collagen implants. Arch Dermatol. 1983;119(6):533–4.
86. Charriere G, Bejot M, Schnitzler L, Ville G, Hartman DJ. Reactions to a bovine collagen implant: clinical and immunologic study in 705 patients. J Am Acad Dermatol. 1989;21(6):1203–8. https://doi.org/10.1016/s0190-9622(89)70330-3.
87. Berke GS, Gerratt B, Kreiman J, Jackson K. Treatment of Parkinson hypophonia with percutaneous collagen augmentation. Laryngoscope. 1999;109(8):1295–9.
88. Sagawa M, Sato M, Fujimura S, Sakurada A, Takahashi H, Kondo T, et al. Vocal fold injection of collagen for unilateral vocal fold paralysis caused by chest diseases. J Cardiovasc Surg. 1999;40(4):603–5.
89. DeVore DP, Hughes E, Scott JB. Effectiveness of injectable filler materials for smoothing wrinkle lines and depressed scars. Med Prog Technol. 1994;20(3–4):243–50.
90. Ford CN, Staskowski PA, Bless DM. Autologous collagen vocal fold injection: a preliminary clinical study. Laryngoscope. 1995;105(9 Pt 1):944–8. https://doi.org/10.1288/00005537-199509000-00014.
91. Remacle M, Lawson G, Delos M, Jamart J. Correcting vocal fold immobility by autologous collagen injection for voice rehabilitation. A short-term study. Ann Otol Rhinol Laryngol. 1999;108(8):788–93. https://doi.org/10.1177/000348949910800813.
92. Remacle M, Lawson G, Keghian J, Jamart J. Use of injectable autologous collagen for correcting glottic gaps: initial results. J Voice. 1999;13(2):280–8. https://doi.org/10.1016/s0892-1997(99)80033-2.
93. Courey MS. Homologous collagen substances for vocal fold augmentation. Laryngoscope. 2001; 111(5):747–58. https://doi.org/10.1097/00005537-200105000-00001.
94. Owens JM. Soft tissue implants and fillers. Otolaryngol Clin N Am. 2005;38(2):361–9. https://doi.org/10.1016/j.otc.2004.10.003.
95. Sengor A, Aydin O, Mola F, Gürbüz Y. Evaluation of alloderm and autologous skin in quadriceps muscles of rats for injection laryngoplasty. Eur Arch Otorhinolaryngol. 2005;262(2):107–12. https://doi.org/10.1007/s00405-004-0756-6.
96. Lundy DS, Casiano RR, McClinton ME, Xue JW. Early results of transcutaneous injection laryngoplasty with micronized acellular dermis versus type-I thyroplasty for glottic incompetence dysphonia due to unilateral vocal fold paralysis. J Voice. 2003;17(4):589–95. https://doi.org/10.1067/s0892-1997(03)00081-x.
97. Karpenko AN, Dworkin JP, Meleca RJ, Stachler RJ. Cymetra injection for unilateral vocal cord paralysis. Ann Otol Rhinol Laryngol. 2003;112(11):927–34. https://doi.org/10.1177/000348940311201103.

Surgical Anatomy for Vocal Fold Injection

2

Sang Hyuk Lee

Abstract

Vocal fold injection (VFI) is a surgical procedure that has gained popularity in the past two decades owing to its technical improvement and clinical efficacy. VFI is made up of injection laryngoplasty for glottic insufficiency and intralesional steroid injection on benign vocal fold (VF) lesions. A variety of approaches are currently available to perform VFI under local anesthesia. Among these introduced methods, transcutaneous injection offers many advantages, but it has some technical difficulties during access to the VF. The purpose of this chapter is to provide a guide to the anatomy of the larynx for better VFI approaches. The initial step of VFI is ascertaining laryngeal landmarks by palpation. The most important landmarks are the thyroid notch, inferior border of the thyroid cartilage, cricoid cartilage, and cricothyroid membrane. It is crucial for the laryngologist to be familiar with the surgical anatomy of larynx and VF in order to improve the accuracy of VFI.

Keywords

Anatomy of larynx · Vocal fold · Vocal fold injection · Injection laryngoplasty
Intralesional steroid injection
Transcutaneous injection

S. H. Lee (✉)
Department of Otolaryngology Head and Neck Surgery, Sungkyunkwan University School of Medicine, Seoul, South Korea

2.1 Laryngeal Framework

2.1.1 Hyoid Bone

The laryngeal framework comprises bone, cartilages, and muscles. Although the hyoid bone is not contained within the larynx, but it's location is associated with vocal fold injection (VFI), therefore it is needed to be discussed at this chapter. The hyoid bone is a horseshoe-shaped bone consisting of a body and greater and lesser horns on each side. It is situated in the anterior midline of the neck, and serves as attachment for numerous muscles of the mouth floor above and some of muscles of the larynx below. It is suspended from the tip of the styloid process of the temporal bone by the stylohyoid ligament and connected with the larynx by the thyrohyoid membrane. The hyoid bone plays an important role including swallowing and speech.

2.1.2 Thyroid Cartilage

Thyroid cartilage is the largest of the laryngeal cartilages, in which located front of the larynx and 1 cm below the hyoid bone. It comprises two quadrilateral halves, which fused in the midline as the laryngeal prominence. The superior border of

© Springer Nature Singapore Pte Ltd. 2021
B.-J. Lee et al. (eds.), *Vocal Fold Injection*, https://doi.org/10.1007/978-981-16-3303-4_2

the laminae meets in the midline as a V-shaped notch, superior thyroid notch. The angle formed at the thyroid notch is more acute in the male than the female. The superior border of the thyroid cartilage is concave and attached to the hyoid bone by the thyrohyoid membrane. And the inferior border is concave posteriorly and convex anteriorly and gives attachment to the cricothyroid ligament. The thyroid cartilage forms a shield of the front wall of the larynx, and protects the vocal folds (VFs), which are located in the middle of the cartilage. The thyroid cartilage ossifies with age, usually begins at approximately 30 years of age. In the elderly, ossification is a lot in progress so VFI through the thyroid cartilage is difficult.

2.1.3 Cricoid Cartilage

The cricoid cartilage is a hyaline cartilage that lies in the inferior-most boundary of the laryngeal skeleton. It is a complete full ring in shape, and has a narrow arch anteriorly which widens into a broad lamina posterior to the airway. Posteriorly, it has a large quadrate-shaped lamina which is 2–3 cm in vertical height [1]. The superior border of the posterior lamina has two small convex facets that serve as the articular surfaces for the arytenoid cartilages. The cricoid's articular facet for the cricothyroid joint is at the point where the lamina narrows to become the arch. The cricothyroid cartilage is usually identifiable by palpating and provides the most constant surface landmark for VFI (Figs. 2.1 and 2.2).

2.2 Laryngeal Membranes and Ligaments

The various parts of the larynx are connected by mucosal folds, ligaments, and membranes. The laryngeal membranes and ligaments support the laryngeal skeleton. The mucosal lining of the larynx is connected with that of the pharynx, and forms several folds. The ligaments and membranes can be divided into extrinsic and intrinsic groups. Extrinsic group attaches the larynx to other structures such as the hyoid bone or the trachea, whereas intrinsic group connects between the laryngeal cartilages (Fig. 2.2).

2.2.1 Extrinsic

The extrinsic group consists of the thyrohyoid, hyoepiglottic, and cricotracheal ligaments. The

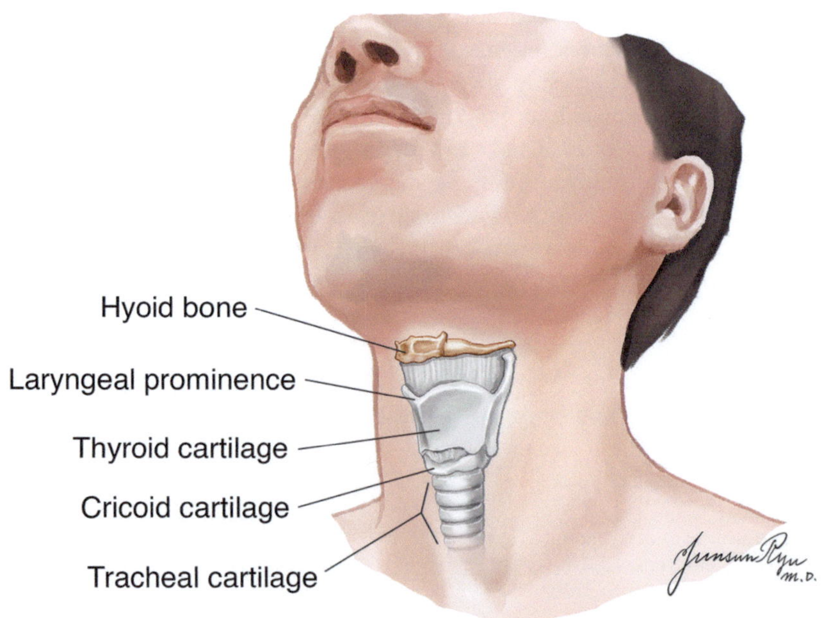

Fig. 2.1 Surface landmarks for vocal fold injection

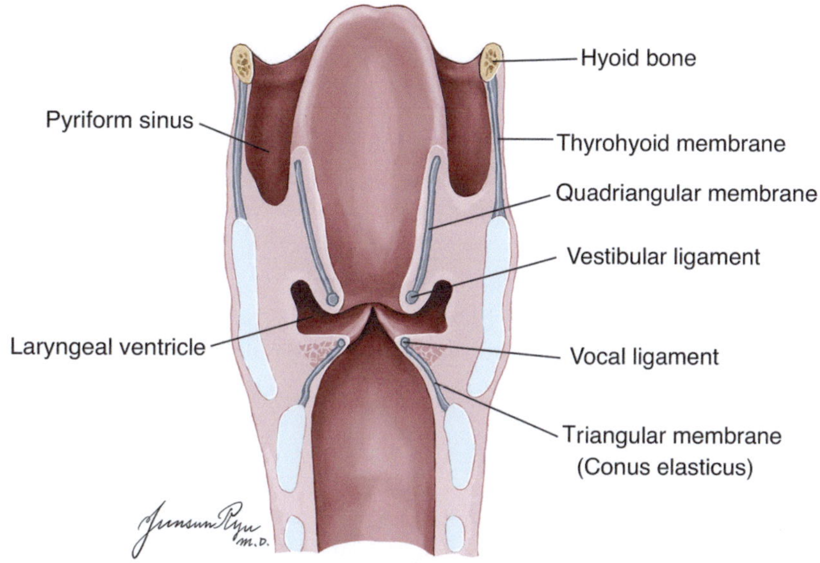

Fig. 2.2 Laryngeal membrane and ligaments

thyrohyoid membrane is a broad fibroelastic membrane and attaches the posterior surface of the body of the hyoid bone and the superior border of the thyroid cartilage. Bilaterally it is thickened as the lateral thyrohyoid ligament, which directly attaches to the superior horn of the thyroid cartilage and in the median region becomes thickened as the median thyrohyoid ligament. The lateral side of the median thyrohyoid ligament is the point where the superior laryngeal vessels and nerve enter the larynx. The hyoepiglottic ligament extends from the midline of the superior surface of the epiglottis to the superior border of the hyoid bone. The cricotracheal ligament connects the cricoid cartilage with the first tracheal ring.

2.2.2 Intrinsic

There are two intrinsic membranes, the quadrangular membrane and the conus elasticus. The quadrangular membranes exist as a pair and connect the epiglottis with the arytenoid and thyroid cartilages. The superior border of the quadrangular membrane descends obliquely from the superior part of the epiglottis to the corniculate cartilage and forms aryepiglottic folds. The inferior border forms the vestibular ligament, which is located in the false VFs. The conus elasticus, also known as the triangular membrane, connects the cricoid cartilage with the thyroid and arytenoid cartilages. It has dense fibroconnective tissue with abundant elastic fibers. There are two components of the conus elasticus, the medial cricothyroid ligament and the lateral cricothyroid membranes. The thick anterior part of the membrane is the medial cricothyroid ligament that connects the anterior part of the arch of the cricoid cartilage with the inferior border of the thyroid membrane. The lateral cricothyroid membrane originates from the superior border of the cricoid arch, rises superiorly and medially and is attached to the vocal process of the arytenoid cartilages posteriorly, and to the internal middle part of the thyroid cartilage anteriorly. Its superior free borders form the vocal ligament and is located in the true VFs. The point where the vocal ligaments attach to the thyroid cartilage is Broyles' tendon. The tendons of both sides covered by the epithelium form the anterior commissure. The lateral cricothyroid membrane also provides attachment to the cricothyroid muscle on each side, as well as to the lateral and posterior crico-arytenoid muscles.

2.3 Laryngeal Cavity

2.3.1 Preepiglottic Space

The preepiglottic space (PES) is an inverted pyramid-shaped space surrounded by the hyoepiglottic ligament superiorly, the thyrohyoid ligament anteriorly, and anterior surface of the epiglottis and the thyroepiglottic ligament posteriorly. The PES is open and continuous with each of the two paraglottic spaces [2].

2.3.2 Paraglottic Space

The paraglottic space (PGS) is situated lateral to the true and false VFs and extends laterally to the thyroid cartilage. PGS is a potential space surrounded by the inner wall of the thyroid cartilage on the outside, conus elasticus inferomedially, laryngeal ventricle medially. Anteriorly, each PGS is continuous with the PES [3]. The mean estimated volume of the preepiglottic and paraglottic space using spiral computed tomography was 2.8 ml (SD 1.7 ml, range 0.7–5.9) [4].

2.4 Vocal Fold

2.4.1 Gross Anatomy

The VFs are located within the larynx at the top of the trachea. They are attached to the arytenoid cartilages posteriorly, and to the thyroid cartilage anteriorly. The level of VF was determined between the thyroid notch and inferior border of the thyroid cartilage [5]. Males and females have different VF sizes. The male VFs are between 1.75 and 2.5 cm while in female VFs are between 1.25 and 1.75 cm in length [6]. The location of the anterior commissure in relation to the height of the anterior midline of the thyroid cartilage is variable. In general, the anterior commissure is located at or above the midpoint of the anterior midline of the thyroid cartilage in women, and it is located below the midpoint in men [7].

2.4.2 Microanatomy

Understanding about the microanatomy of VF is also required to determine the target of injection. The VFs are very complex multilayered structures suitable for phonation. Medially to laterally, the membranous VF consists of squamous epithelium, Reinke's space (superficial layer of the lamina propria), the vocal ligament (intermediate and deep layer of the lamina propria), and the thyroarytenoid muscle. (Figs. 2.2 and 2.3) The epithelium of VFs consists of a pseudostratified ciliated columnar epithelium that promotes mucus secretion. The epithelial layer of VFs is very thin and helps maintain the shape of VFs. The thickness of the Reinke's space is about 0.3 mm and is mainly composed of loose fibers and substrates. It consists of collagen, which is rich in fluidity, and is important for phonation through vigorous vibration of the VF mucosa. The Reinke's space is a region that is easily damaged by excessive stimulation or vocalization.

The vocal ligament is made up of elastin and collagen fibers. Elastin fibers impart the elasticity to the VFs and can be stretched up to about five times their original size. These fibers are concentrated in the vocal ligament, especially in the intermediate layer of the lamina propria [8]. Collagen fibers are responsible for the resistance and elasticity to tensile strength, and balance the tension in the lamina propria, thus allowing the vocal ligament to stand the tension of the intrinsic muscle of the larynx during phonation [9]. These fibers are concentrated in the deep layer of the lamina propria [10, 11]. In the muscular layer, the medial portions of the thyroarytenoid are called vocalis muscle, and these muscle fibers are located parallel to the vocal ligament.

In VF steroid injection, care should be taken to inject into the superficial layer of lamina propria not deeper than the vocal ligament in order not to affect thyroarytenoid muscle activity [12]. VF steroid injection may induced muscular or submucosal glandular atrophy in a few cases, which was self-limited in animal study [13]. For medialization VFI, when the material injected into the submucosa of the VFs, it may damage the viscoelasticity of the VF mucosa, so care should be taken not to inject into the superficial layer of the VFs [14].

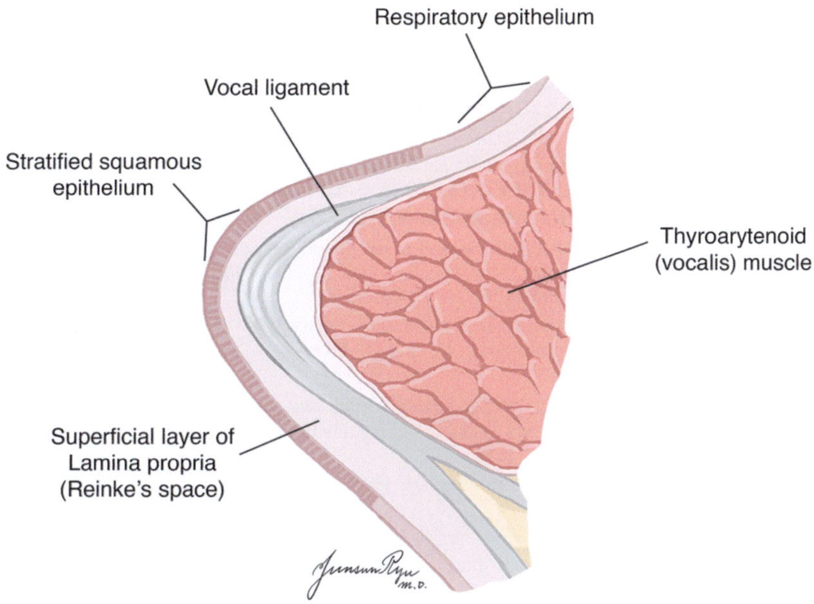

Fig. 2.3 Cross section of the vocal fold

2.5 Anatomical Consideration for VFI

The initial step for percutaneous VFI is ascertaining laryngeal surface landmarks by palpation. The most important landmarks are the thyroid notch, inferior border of thyroid cartilage and cricoid cartilage. The cricothyroid membrane is palpable as the dip between inferior to the thyroid cartilage and superior to the cricoid cartilage. However, it might be difficult to identify the landmark by palpation especially in patients with a short and wide neck and a history of neck surgery or radiation therapy. Special cautions are needed as the anatomical indicators of the normal neck may be distorted. In transcutaneous VFI, needle tip need to be estimated through laryngoscope while moving the needle, so much understanding of the laryngeal anatomy is required.

Transcutaneous injection via cricothyroid membrane is approached from the surface at the inferior margin of the thyroid cartilage, 3–7 mm lateral to the midline through the cricothyroid membrane, and subsequently passed cephalad and laterally. In a cadaver study, thickness of the cricothyroid membrane was 3.54 mm in males, 2.70 mm in females [15] and 4.53 mm in males, 2.89 mm in females [16]. The average length from the lower edge of the thyroid cartilage to the VFs is 15.14 mm in males and 13.60 mm in females [17]. For the trans-thyrohyoid membrane approach, the needle is inserted immediately above the thyrohyoid notch and through the subcutaneous tissues at a downward angle, passing though the preepiglottic space and entering the larynx at the level of the petiole of the epiglottis [18].

Key Learning Points:

- After appropriate positioning of neck partially extended, surface neck landmarks (hyoid bone, thyroid cartilage, and cricoid cartilage) need to be confirmed by palpation.
- Superior thyroid notch and cricoid cartilage provides the most constant surface landmark for VFI.
- The cricothyroid membrane is identifiable by first palpating the anterior portion of the cricoid cartilage and by superiorly palpating the inferior border of thyroid cartilage.
- Although, there is some individual diversity concerning the thicknesses of skin and subcutaneous tissues, the distance from skin to VFs via the cricothyroid membrane usually measured within 2 cm.

References

1. Fried M, Meller S, Rinaldo A. Adult laryngeal anatomy. The Larynx. 1988;2
2. Sato K, Kurita S, Hirano M. Location of the preepiglottic space and its relationship to the paraglottic space. Ann Otol Rhinol Laryngol. 1993;102(12):930–4.
3. Watkinson J, Gilbert R. Stell & Maran's textbook of head and neck surgery and oncology. New York: CRC; 2011.
4. Hermans R, Van der Goten A, Baert A. Volume estimation of the preepiglottic and paraglottic space using spiral computed tomography. Surg Radiol Anat. 1997;19(3):185–8.
5. Flint PW, et al. Cummings otolaryngology-head and neck surgery e-book. New York: Elsevier Health Sciences; 2014.
6. Titze IR. Principles of voice production. Englewood Cliffs: Prentice Hall; 1994.
7. Cinar U, et al. Level of vocal folds as projected on the exterior thyroid cartilage. Laryngoscope. 2003;113(10):1813–6.
8. Hammond TH, et al. Age-and gender-related elastin distribution changes in human vocal folds: student research award 1997. Otolaryngol Head Neck Surg. 1998;119(4):314–22.
9. Gray SD, et al. Biomechanical and histologic observations of vocal fold fibrous proteins. Ann Otol Rhinol Laryngol. 2000;109(1):77–85.
10. <distribution of collagen in the lamina propria of the human vocal fold.pdf>.
11. Sato K, Hirano M, Nakashima T. Age-related changes of collagenous fibers in the human vocal fold mucosa. Ann Otol Rhinol Laryngol. 2002;111(1):15–20.
12. Wang CT, et al. Intralesional steroid injection for benign vocal fold disorders: a systematic review and meta-analysis. Laryngoscope. 2013;123(1):197–203.
13. Jin HJ, et al. Morphological and histological changes of rabbit vocal fold after steroid injection. Otolaryngol Head Neck Surg. 2013;149(2):277–83.
14. Rosen CA. Phonosurgical vocal fold injection: procedures and materials. Otolaryngol Clin N Am. 2000;33(5):1087–96.
15. Prithishkumar IJ, David SS. Morphometric analysis and clinical application of the working dimensions of cricothyroid membrane in south Indian adults: with special relevance to surgical cricothyroidotomy. Emerg Med Australas. 2010;22(1):13–20.
16. Anand V, et al. Surgical anatomy of cricothyroid membrane with reference to airway surgeries in north Indian population: a cadaveric study. Int J Otorhinolaryngol Head Neck Surg. 2018;4
17. Jin SM, et al. Transcutaneous injection laryngoplasty through the cricothyroid space in the sitting position: anatomical information and technique. Eur Arch Otorhinolaryngol. 2008;265(3):313–9.
18. Amin MR. Thyrohyoid approach for vocal fold augmentation. Ann Otol Rhinol Laryngol. 2006;115(9):699–702.

3 Indications for Vocal Fold Injection

Joo Hyun Woo

Abstract

Vocal fold injection (VFI) was introduced as a treatment of unilateral vocal fold paralysis (UVFP). In recent years, the range of indications for VFI is widening. Vocal fold botulinum toxin injection is the treatment of choice for the spasmodic dysphonia, and vocal fold steroid injection is alternatively used for the treatment of the benign vocal fold lesions.

Keywords

Vocal fold injection · Vocal fold paralysis
Glottic insufficiency · Spasmodic dysphonia
Benign vocal fold lesions

3.1 Unilateral Vocal Fold Paralysis

3.1.1 Definition

Unilateral vocal fold paralysis (UVFP) occurs due to the loss of innervation of the recurrent laryngeal nerve (RLN) and results in voice change of various degrees [1].

J. H. Woo (✉)
Department of Otorhinolaryngology-Head and Neck Surgery, College of Medicine, Gachon University, Incheon, South Korea
e-mail: woojh@gilhospital.com

3.1.2 Etiology

3.1.2.1 Iatrogenic

The unilateral vocal fold paralysis (UVFP) occurs when the recurrent laryngeal nerve (RLN) or the vagus nerve is pulled, severed, or damaged by a heating device during operation such as thyroidectomy, cervical disc surgery via anterior approach, esophagectomy, cardiothoracic surgery, and neck dissection [2]. Although rare, vocal fold paralysis is possible due to endotracheal intubation, which requires discrimination from dislocation of the arytenoid cartilage [3].

3.1.2.2 Neoplastic (Non Laryngeal)

The tumor may invade the RLN or the vagus nerve, resulting in UVFP. Lung cancer is the most common cause of tumor invasion, and in addition, esophageal cancer, thyroid cancer, and low-cranial tumors are also possible too [4].

3.1.2.3 Idiopathic

It is diagnosed as idiopathic when the cause is not identified in several diagnostic tests including detailed medical history, laryngoscopic examination, and imaging studies [3].

3.1.3 Evaluation

3.1.3.1 History Taking

History taking about the patient's symptoms, duration of symptoms, past medical history, and

© Springer Nature Singapore Pte Ltd. 2021

B.-J. Lee et al. (eds.), *Vocal Fold Injection*, https://doi.org/10.1007/978-981-16-3303-4_3

surgical history can be important data in inferring the cause of UVFP, conducting an examination, and deciding treatment.

3.1.3.2 Laryngoscopy and Stroboscopy

Laryngoscopy is an essential test for identifying impairment of vocal fold movement [4]. In laryngoscopy, repeating/i/and sniff can maximize the vocal fold movement to further clarify the motility [5]. Stroboscope can evaluate not only movement disorders of the vocal folds, but also glottic insufficiency, height difference between both vocal folds, and asymmetry of mucosal wave [6].

3.1.3.3 Imaging Studies

Neck CT or magnetic resonance imaging (MRI) encompassing an area from the skull base to the superior mediastinum is necessary to rule out the neoplastic etiology of UVFP [7].

3.1.3.4 Voice Assessments

Voice assessments, such as perception, acoustics, aerodynamics, and self-rating questionnaires are necessary to define treatment goal and provide visual feedback to clinicians and patients, before and after management of UVFP [7].

3.1.3.5 Laryngeal Electromyography

Laryngeal electromyography can help predict the prognosis of UVFP and differentiate it from mechanical disorders such as fixation or dislocation of the cricoarytenoid joint [8].

3.1.4 Treatment

3.1.4.1 Principle

The goals of treatment for UVFP are to improve hoarseness and prevent aspiration. There are several options for treatments, such as waiting spontaneous recovery, voice therapy, and surgery. When selecting a treatment method, the patient's voice demand, the presence or absence of aspiration, the prevalence period of UVFP, the wideness of glottic gap, and the possibility of spontaneous recovery should be carefully considered.

3.1.4.2 Spontaneous Recovery

If it is not clear that the nerve has been severed, the vocal cord motility can be restored spontaneously, so follow-up observation is possible for 6–12 months [9–11].

3.1.4.3 Voice Therapy

The effect of voice therapy in UVFP is to improve glottic closure using appropriate compensatory mechanism [12]. Voice therapy may be improve voice outcomes for the patient with mild symptoms. Also pre and post-operative voice therapy is helpful for optimal postoperative phonation [13].

3.1.4.4 Surgical Management

Vocal fold injection (VFI), medialization thyroplasty, arytenoid adduction, and reinnervation are available as surgical treatment in UVFP [14, 15].

3.2 Benign Vocal Fold Lesions

3.2.1 Definition

Although there is no consensus about the definition for Benign vocal fold lesions (BVFLs), BVFLs are known as tumor- like lesions caused by an inflammatory reaction of the vocal folds including nodules, polyps, cysts, fibrous masses, and pseudocysts [16]. They are located in lamina propria and thereby interrupt the mucosal wave of vocal folds. Among BVFLs, vocal nodule, vocal polyp and Reinke's edema are frequently encountered in clinics. Although pathological examination reveals subtle differences between these lesions, most present as phonotrauma, chronic inflammation, and subsequent remodeling of the superficial lamina propria [17, 18].

3.2.2 Etiology

Although the cause of BVFLs is controversial, voice abuse, cigarette smoking, and laryngoesophageal reflux are considered as causative factors for BVFLs [19]. Voice abuse and overuse cause repetitive damage to the vocal fold mucosa [20].

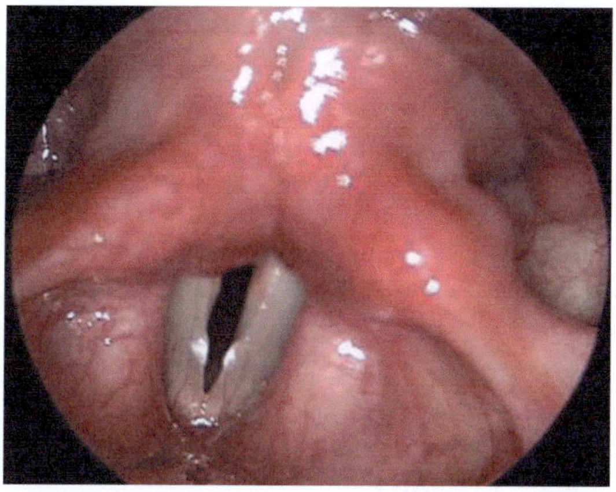

Fig. 3.1 Vocal nodules. There are whitish nodular lesions in the middle of the bilateral vocal folds

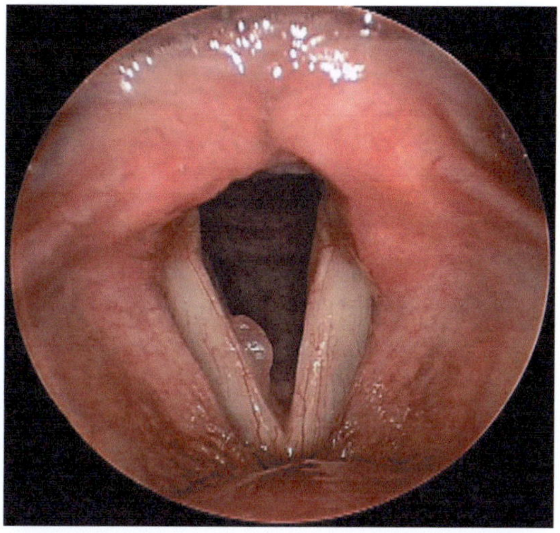

Fig. 3.2 Vocal polyp. In the right vocal fold, a translucent polyp with broad attachment rather than pedunculated attachment is found

Cigarette smoking induces chronic irritation to the vocal fold mucosa and alters permeability of capillary walls leading to extravasation of fluid into Reinke's space, and subsequently makes vocal fold swelling [21]. Laryngoesophageal reflux induce mucus modification, epithelial ulceration and microtrauma, muscular hyperfunctional effect, and Reinke's space dryness in vocal fold [19, 22].

3.2.3 Diagnosis

BVFLs can often be diagnosed by their appearance during laryngoscopy and stroboscopy [23]. Vocal nodules appear mainly bilaterally in the form of protruding white thickened epithelium in the middle of the vocal folds (Fig. 3.1). Mucosal waves are normal or slightly reduced [24]. Vocal polyp mainly occurs in unilateral vocal fold and are visually observed as translucent mucous or angiomatous mass (Fig. 3.2) [25]. In Reinke's edema, both vocal folds looks like spindle-shape gelatin pockets caused by lymphatic retention and venous congestion in Reinke's space (Fig. 3.3).

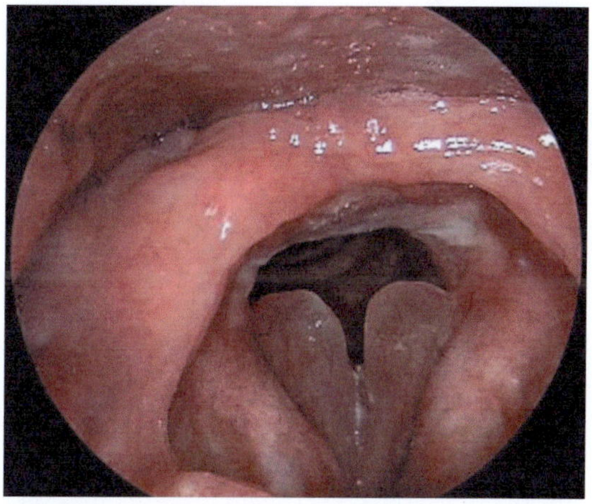

Fig. 3.3 Reinke's edema. Diffuse pale polypoid change is presented in both vocal folds

3.2.4 Treatment

Currently, standard treatments for BVFLs include voice hygiene, voice therapy, and laryngeal microsurgery [26]. Although laryngeal microsurgery is preferred as the initial treatment for vocal polyp, voice hygiene education and vocie therapy should be basically performed in the treatment of BVFLs [27, 28]. However, if they are not effective or not available be performed, vocal fold steroid injection could be used as an adjustive method [27, 29, 30].

3.3 Spasmodic Dysphonia

3.3.1 Definition

Spasmodic dysphonia (SD) is recognized as a task-specific focal laryngal dystonia characterized by irregular and uncontrolled voice breaks accompaning by effortful phonation [31]. It is most prevalent in middle-aged women [32]. Clear classification is difficult, but there are two types of SD: adductor spasmodic dysphonia (AdSD), characterized by a harsh, strain-strangled voice with breaks on vowels in speech, and abductor spasmodic dysphonia (AbSD), characterized by prolonged voiceless consonants before vowels [33, 34].

3.3.2 Etiology

Traditionally, spasmodic dysphonia was thought to result from basal ganglia abnormalities, but the pathophysiology of SD has not been clearly identified [31]. Currently, SD is considered as a complex disorder likely due to a multifactorial etiology, including neurological, genetic, and environmental factors [35].

3.3.3 Diagnosis

The diagnosis of spasmodic dysphonia can be difficult due to the lack of a scientific consensus on diagnostic criteria [36]. Clinical diagnosis depends on voice care teams including otolaryngologists, speech-language pathologists (SLP), and neurologists experienced in the identification and treatment of SD, voice tremor, and muscular tension dysphonia [37]. SD usually does not respond to voice therapy alone. SD also tends to be task dependent, meaning that the severity of voice symptoms can vary with specific speech sounds [36]. Visualization of the larynx by laryngoscopy is needed to exclude other laryngeal abnormalities such as vocal fold paralysis [37].

3.3.4 Treatment

The current gold standard of therapy is the administration of botulinum toxin injection in the adductor musculature, causing a temporary chemical denervation of the injected adductors resulting in an incomplete glottic closure by a paresis of the vocal fold [38].

3.4 Vocal Process Granuloma

3.4.1 Definition

Vocal process granuloma (VPG) is benign, hypertrophic granulation tissue located on the medial surface of the vocal process of the arytenoid cartilage [39]. VPG is more common in male than in female. It can also occur in pediatrics, but mainly in adults [40].

3.4.2 Etiology

Several etiological factors have been suggested, such as intubation trauma, hard glottal attack, vocal misuse, laryngopharyngeal reflux (LPR), habitual throat clearing, low-pitched voice, and psychosomatic disorders [41, 42]. Smoking, postnasal drip, and throat infections may also be associated with VPG.

3.4.3 Diagnosis

Laryngoscopy typically exposes an image of vocal process granuloma as either an ulcerated or space occupying lesion [40]. contact granuloma is mainly unilateral, (Fig. 3.4) though intubation granuloma is usually bilateral.

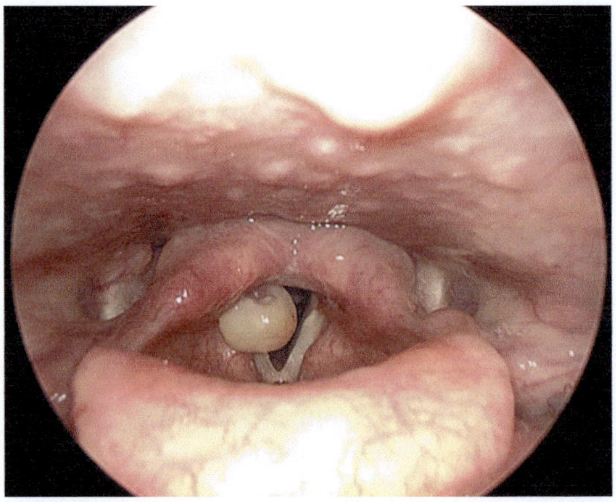

Fig. 3.4 Contact granuloma. There is a round granulomatous mass on right vocal process

3.4.4 Treatment

Voice therapy and proton pump inhibitor are known as primary treatments for VPG. However, in the refractory case for primary treatment, botulium toxin injection into the affected vocal fold is recommended as the most effective treatment [43–45]. Surgery reserved only for failures of medical treatment or airway obstruction or when diagnosis is in doubt [45].

Key Learning Points:

- VFI is one of the primary treatment options for UVFP.
- Vocal fold steroid injection can be considered for the treatment of BVFLs such as vocal nodule, vocal poly, and Reinke's edema.
- Vocal fold botulinum toxin injection can be expected to have a good therapeutic effect in spasmodic dysphonia and refractory vocal process granuloma.

References

1. Walton C, Conway E, Blackshaw H, Carding P. Unilateral vocal fold paralysis: a systematic review of speech-language pathology management. J Voice. 2017;31(4):509.
2. Misono S, Merati AL. Evidence-based practice: evaluation and management of unilateral vocal fold paralysis. Otolaryngol Clin N Am. 2012;45(5):1083–108.
3. Rosenthal LH, Benninger MS, Deeb RH. Vocal fold immobility: a longitudinal analysis of etiology over 20 years. Laryngoscope. 2007;117(10):1864–70.
4. Benninger MS, Crumley RL, Ford CN, Gould WJ, Hanson DG, Ossoff RH, et al. Evaluation and treatment of the unilateral paralyzed vocal fold. Otolaryngol Head Neck Surg. 1994;111(4):497–508.
5. Rubin AD, Praneetvatakul V, Heman-Ackah Y, Moyer CA, Mandel S, Sataloff RT. Repetitive phonatory tasks for identifying vocal fold paresis. J Voice. 2005;19(4):679–86.
6. Bonilha HS, Desjardins M, Garand KL, Martin-Harris B. Parameters and scales used to assess and report findings from Stroboscopy: a systematic review. J Voice. 2018;32(6):734–55.
7. Ryu CH, Kwon TK, Kim H, Kim HS, Park IS, Woo JH, et al. Guidelines for the management of unilateral vocal fold paralysis from the Korean Society of Laryngology, Phoniatrics and Logopedics. Clin Exp Otorhinolaryngol. 2020; https://doi.org/10.21053/ceo.2020.00409.
8. Blitzer A, Crumley RL, Dailey SH, Ford CN, Floeter MK, Hillel AD, et al. Recommendations of the Neurolaryngology Study Group on laryngeal electromyography. Otolaryngol Head Neck Surg. 2009;140(6):782–93.
9. Jeannon JP, Orabi AA, Bruch GA, Abdalsalam HA, Simo R. Diagnosis of recurrent laryngeal nerve palsy after thyroidectomy: a systematic review. Int J Clin Pract. 2009;63(4):624–9.
10. Chen X, Wan P, Yu Y, Li M, Xu Y, Huang P, et al. Types and timing of therapy for vocal fold paresis/paralysis after thyroidectomy: a systematic review and meta-analysis. J Voice. 2014;28(6):799–808.
11. Sulica L. The natural history of idiopathic unilateral vocal fold paralysis: evidence and problems. Laryngoscope. 2008;118(7):1303–7.
12. Rubin AD, Sataloff RT. Vocal fold paresis and paralysis. Otolaryngol Clin N Am. 2007;40(5):1109–31. viii-ix
13. Isshiki N. Mechanical and dynamic aspects of voice production as related to voice therapy and phonosurgery. Otolaryngol Head Neck Surg. 2000;122(6):782–93.
14. Granato F, Martelli F, Comini LV, Luparello P, Coscarelli S, Le Seac O, et al. The surgical treatment of unilateral vocal cord paralysis (UVCP): qualitative review analysis and meta-analysis study. Eur Arch Otorhinolaryngol. 2019;276(10):2649–59.
15. Siu J, Tam S, Fung K. A comparison of outcomes in interventions for unilateral vocal fold paralysis: a systematic review. Laryngoscope. 2016;126(7):1616–24.
16. Anis MM, Memon Z. Injection medialization laryngoplasty improves dysphagia in patients with unilateral vocal fold immobility. World J Otorhinolaryngol Head Neck Surg. 2018;4(2):126–9.
17. Wang CT, Liao LJ, Cheng PW, Lo WC, Lai MS. Intralesional steroid injection for benign vocal fold disorders: a systematic review and meta-analysis. Laryngoscope. 2013;123(1):197–203.
18. Wallis L, Jackson-Menaldi C, Holland W, Giraldo A. Vocal fold nodule vs. vocal fold polyp: answer from surgical pathologist and voice pathologist point of view. J Voice. 2004;18(1):125–9.
19. Lechien JR, Saussez S, Nacci A, Barillari MR, Rodriguez A, Le Bon SD, et al. Association between laryngopharyngeal reflux and benign vocal folds lesions: a systematic review. Laryngoscope. 2019;129(9):E329–e41.
20. Birchall MA, Carding P. Vocal nodules management. Clin Otolaryngol. 2019;44(4):497–501.
21. Tan M, Bryson PC, Pitts C, Woo P, Benninger MS. Clinical grading of Reinke's edema. Laryngoscope. 2017;127(10):2310–3.
22. Lechien JR, Saussez S, Harmegnies B, Finck C, Burns JA. Laryngopharyngeal reflux and voice disorders: a multifactorial model of etiology and pathophysiology. J Voice. 2017;31(6):733–52.

23. Naunheim MR, Carroll TL. Benign vocal fold lesions: update on nomenclature, cause, diagnosis, and treatment. Curr Opin Otolaryngol Head Neck Surg. 2017;25(6):453–8.
24. Rosen CA, Gartner-Schmidt J, Hathaway B, Simpson CB, Postma GN, Courey M, et al. A nomenclature paradigm for benign midmembranous vocal fold lesions. Laryngoscope. 2012;122(6):1335–41.
25. Kantas I, Balatsouras DG, Kamargianis N, Katotomichelakis M, Riga M, Danielidis V. The influence of laryngopharyngeal reflux in the healing of laryngeal trauma. Eur Arch Otorhinolaryngol. 2009;266(2):253–9.
26. Hosoya M, Kobayashi R, Ishii T, Senarita M, Kuroda H, Misawa H, et al. Vocal hygiene education program reduces surgical interventions for benign vocal fold lesions: a randomized controlled trial. Laryngoscope. 2018;128(11):2593–9.
27. Lee SW, Park KN. Long-term efficacy of percutaneous steroid injection for treating benign vocal fold lesions: a prospective study. Laryngoscope. 2016;126(10):2315–9.
28. Wang H, Zhuge P, You H, Zhang Y, Zhang Z. Comparison of the efficacy of vocal training and vocal microsurgery in patients with early vocal fold polyp. Braz J Otorhinolaryngol. 2019;85(6):678–84.
29. Wang CT, Lai MS, Cheng PW. Long-term surveillance following Intralesional steroid injection for benign vocal fold lesions. JAMA Otolaryngol Head Neck Surg. 2017;143(6):589–94.
30. Shoffel-Havakuk H, Sadoughi B, Sulica L, Johns MM 3rd. In-office procedures for the treatment of benign vocal fold lesions in the awake patient: a contemporary review. Laryngoscope. 2019;129(9):2131–8.
31. Whurr R, Lorch M. Review of differential diagnosis and management of spasmodic dysphonia. Current Curr Opin Otolaryngol Head Neck Surg. 2016;24(3):203–7.
32. Schweinfurth JM, Billante M, Courey MS. Risk factors and demographics in patients with spasmodic dysphonia. Laryngoscope. 2002;112(2):220–3.
33. Sapienza CM, Walton S, Murry T. Acoustic variations in adductor spasmodic dysphonia as a function of speech task. J Speech Lang Hear Res. 1999;42(1):127–40.
34. Edgar JD, Sapienza CM, Bidus K, Ludlow CL. Acoustic measures of symptoms in abductor spasmodic dysphonia. J Voice. 2001;15(3):362–72.
35. Hintze JM, Ludlow CL, Bansberg SF, Adler CH, Lott DG. Spasmodic dysphonia: a review. Part 1: pathogenic factors. Otolaryngol Head Neck Surg. 2017;157(4):551–7.
36. Hintze JM, Ludlow CL, Bansberg SF, Adler CH, Lott DG. Spasmodic dysphonia: a review. Part 2: characterization of pathophysiology. Otolaryngol Head Neck Surg. 2017;157(4):558–64.
37. Ludlow CL, Domangue R, Sharma D, Jinnah HA, Perlmutter JS, Berke G, et al. Consensus-Based Attributes for Identifying Patients With Spasmodic Dysphonia and Other Voice Disorders. JAMA Otolaryngol Head Neck Surg. 2018;144(8):657–65.
38. Novakovic D, Waters HH, D'Elia JB, Blitzer A. Botulinum toxin treatment of adductor spasmodic dysphonia: longitudinal functional outcomes. Laryngoscope. 2011;121(3):606–12.
39. Tsai SW, Ma YF, Shih LC, Tsou YA, Sung CK. Operative and conservative management of laryngeal contact granuloma: a network analysis and systematic review. J Voice. 2019;S0892-1997(19)30106–7. doi: https://doi.org/10.1016/j.jvoice.2019.08.019.
40. Devaney KO, Rinaldo A, Ferlito A. Vocal process granuloma of the larynx-recognition, differential diagnosis and treatment. Oral Oncol. 2005;41(7):666–9.
41. Kobayashi R, Tsunoda K, Ueha R, Fujimaki Y, Nito T, Yamasoba T. Role of lifestyle modifications for patients with laryngeal granuloma caused by gastro-esophageal reflux: comparison between conservative treatment and the surgical approach. Acta Otolaryngol. 2017;137(3):306–9.
42. Jang M, Basa K, Levi J. Risk factors for laryngeal trauma and granuloma formation in pediatric intubations. Int J Pediatr Otorhinolaryngol. 2018;107:45–52.
43. Lee SW, Hong HJ, Choi SH, Sun DI, Park YH, Lee BJ, et al. Comparison of treatment modalities for contact granuloma: a nationwide multicenter study. Laryngoscope. 2014;124(5):1187–91.
44. Damrose EJ, Damrose JF. Botulinum toxin as adjunctive therapy in refractory laryngeal granuloma. J Laryngol Otol. 2008;122(8):824–8.
45. Karkos PD, George M, Van Der Veen J, Atkinson H, Dwivedi RC, Kim D, et al. Vocal process granulomas: a systematic review of treatment. Ann Otol Rhinol Laryngol. 2014;123(5):314–20.

4 Anesthesia for Vocal Fold Injection

Han Su Kim

Abstract

Office-based vocal fold injections under local anesthesia are frequently performed. Visual guide under laryngoscopy provides precise injection to proper site. The video laryngoscope is passed through the mouth or the nose of the patient. For preventing gag reflex by laryngoscopy and providing more comfortable procedure, anesthesia should be provided to nasal cavity, pharynx, and larynx. Topical lidocaine is most widely used medication on office-based procedure. Lidocaine has short onset time, sufficient duration of action, and wide safety margin of dosage.

The amount of topical and local anesthetics used in injection laryngoplasty rarely exceeds toxic doses, it may cause discomfort, pain, stinging sensation, nausea, unpleasant taste, globus sensation, dysphasia, or dyspnea. The physician should know proper anesthesia techniques and must be familiar with the safe dose and complication of all anesthetics used.

Keywords

Anesthesia · Laryngoplasty · Lidocaine
Oxymetazoline · Nasal decongestants
Office-based procedures

4.1 Introduction

Vocal fold injection was first introduced by Brünning in 1911 as a treatment for unilateral vocal fold immobility. Although historically, the procedure has been performed under general anesthesia via the trans-oral approach, it is now routine to perform vocal fold injection in the office-based procedure with local anesthesia and transcutaneous injection [1].

Visual guide under laryngoscopy is mandatory during office-based injection laryngoplasty. The images from video laryngoscopy should be displayed on a monitor for the clinician, patient, and others to view at the time of the procedure; it can also be recorded. Images are magnified when displayed on the monitor, allowing for precise injection to proper site. Video laryngoscopy is the premise of vocal fold injection. The video laryngoscope is passed through the mouth (rigid) or the nose (flexible fiber-optic laryngoscopy, FFL) of the patient, into the pharynx, and positioned just above the vocal folds. For preventing gag reflex by laryngoscopy and providing more comfortable procedure, anesthesia should be provided

H. S. Kim (✉)
Department of Otolaryngology Head and Neck Surgery, College of Medicine, Ewha Womans University, Seoul, South Korea
e-mail: sevent@ewha.ac.kr

© Springer Nature Singapore Pte Ltd. 2021

B.-J. Lee et al. (eds.), *Vocal Fold Injection*, https://doi.org/10.1007/978-981-16-3303-4_4

to the following three regions, nasal cavity, pharynx, and larynx, before and during the procedure.

Many studies have not conclusively demonstrated a benefit with any anesthetic use in office based endoscopy. Some studies show that the use of topical anesthesia and vasoconstriction within the "nose" before flexible naso-endoscopy provides no significant advantage over the use of no nasal preparation [2–5]. However, it is very discomfort and unpleasant procedure to do injection into the vocal fold without any preparation for the "throat" and the "larynx." Therefore, the physician should know proper anesthesia techniques and also must be familiar with the safe dose and complication of all anesthetics used.

4.2 Anatomy

For preventing gag reflex, anesthesia should be provided to the following three regions (nasal cavity, oropharynx, and larynx) depending on the nerve supply before and during the procedure (Fig. 4.1).

4.2.1 Nasal Cavity

The anterior ethmoidal nerve from the nasociliary nerve (CN 5) supplies the anterior one third of the nasal septum and the nares. The posterior two thirds of the nasal septum and the turbinate are innervated from the greater palatine nerve and lesser palatine nerves from the pterygopalatine ganglion via the maxillary division of the trigeminal nerve (CN 5) (Fig. 4.2) [6].

4.2.2 Oropharynx

The "gag reflex" is triggered by the afferent branch of glossopharyngeal nerve (cranial nerve 9), the main sensory nerve of the oropharynx [7]. Lingual branch innervates the posterior one third of the tongue, vallecula, and anterior surface of epiglottis. Pharyngeal branch innervates the lateral and posterior walls of the pharynx. Tonsillar branch innervates the tonsillar pillars and soft palate [8].

4.2.3 Larynx

Vagal nerve (CN 10) innervates structures beyond epiglottis. The internal branch of superior laryngeal nerve (SLN) provides sensory innervations the laryngeal mucosa just above the vocal folds. The external branch of SLN supplies motor innervation of the cricothyroid muscle. Recurrent laryngeal nerve (RLN) provides sensory innervations below the vocal folds and trachea and motor supply to all the intrinsic laryngeal muscles except cricothyroid muscles [8].

4.3 Medications

As a preparation for FFL, a local anesthetic and/or a decongestant are usually applied to nasal cavity in order to alleviate the nasal pain, and to widen the field of view [9]. Application of decongestant and anesthetic sprays together seems to be the best method of pharmacological preparation of patients for FFL [9]. Meanwhile, topical anesthetic spray to the oropharynx and the larynx is usually applied for preventing gag reflex and cough reflex.

4.3.1 Anesthetics

Various different topical agents; lidocaine, prilocaine, ropivacaine, and bupivacaine have been used in the office-based procedures. The main considerations in the clinical use of anesthetic agents are potency, duration of anesthesia, the speed of onset, and maximum dose. Potency is determined by the lipid solubility of the agent. Less potent local anesthetics must be given in higher concentration and larger doses [7]. Topical lidocaine and prilocaine applications were found to be more efficacious and fast acting medications for anesthesia of the intranasal mucosa compared with bupivacaine, ropivacaine, and saline solution solutions [10].

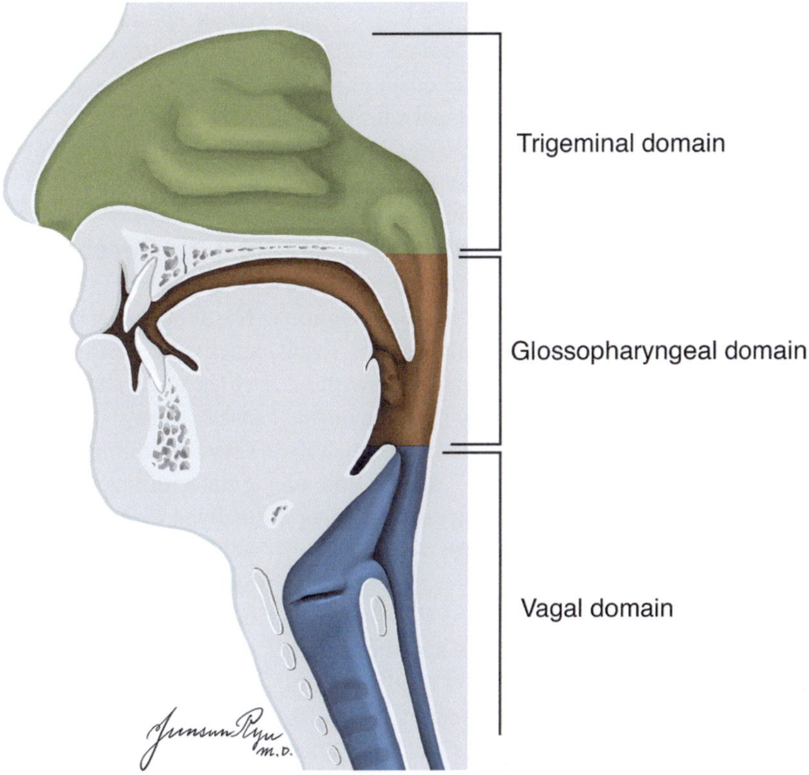

Fig. 4.1 Three domains for local anesthesia for vocal fold injection. The upper airway is divided into three regions depending on its major sensory innervations

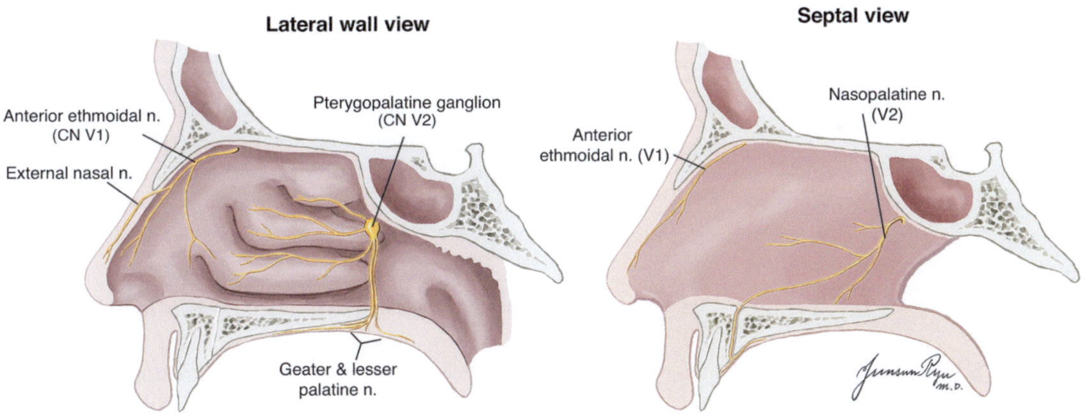

Fig. 4.2 Innervation of the nasal cavity

Lidocaine and tetracaine are the two most commonly used topically applied nasal anesthetics available in a spray form. One study shows that in patients undergoing FFL, use of either 2% tetracaine or 4% lidocaine, has similar effect. Tetracaine may be a better choice in older patients, however, as it was associated with less discomfort, unpleasant taste, globus sensation, and dyspnea [3]. Anesthetic agents are available in different concentrations for topical use (e.g., lidocaine, 4%; tetracaine, 2%). Many such preparations are available commercially in combination with decongestants.

4.3.1.1 Lidocaine

Lidocaine has a low to intermediate potency, 45–60 min duration of action, and onset of sufficient anesthesia within 90 s of topical administration. Lidocaine solutions can be found in 1%, 2%, 4%, and 10% solutions [7]. A 10% lidocaine spray is usually used in office-based procedure and contains 100 mg/mL of lidocaine (Fig. 4.3). About 10 mg of lidocaine is administered on a single spray of 10% lidocaine. The maximum dose of lidocaine "injection" allowed for local infiltration in adults is 4.5 mg/kg/dose without epinephrine and 7 mg/kg/dose with epinephrine [11]. A 70-kg patient can receive approximately 300 mg of lidocaine. "Topical" application of lidocaine for the purpose of office-based procedures rarely exceeds the toxic dose.

4.3.1.2 Tetracaine

Tetracaine is a highly potent local anesthetic with duration of anesthesia between 60 and 120 min when applied topically [7]. It seems to establish the anesthesia of the nasal passage faster than lidocaine. Furthermore, as topical nasal anesthesia, tetracaine has demonstrated superiority to cocaine and lidocaine both in terms of duration of action and pain control [12]. Significant tetracaine associated toxicity has not been reported when applied topically through the nose; however, it is recommended to use less than 1 mL of 2% tetracaine for nasal anesthesia. Typically, only 0.1–0.2 mL is needed when delivered through an atomizer [7].

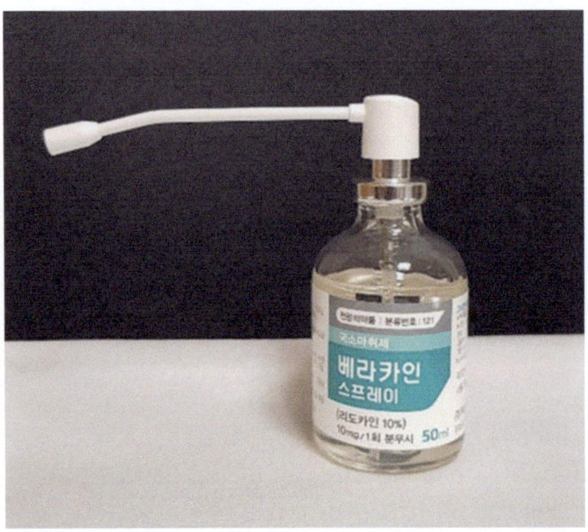

Fig. 4.3 10% lidocaine spray. It contains 100 mg/ml lidocaine. For anesthesia of the throat, larynx, and trachea, the safety dose of this lidocaine spray is up to 200 mg (twenty times of spray)

4.3.2 Decongestants

Nasal decongestants are used for widening nasal cavity by constriction of nasal mucosa. It provides wide nasal passage. The most commonly used drug for this is oxymetazoline. Oxymetazoline is considered to have similar or greater efficacy and less toxicity (hypertension, tachycardia) compared with phenylephrine, epinephrine, and cocaine [13]. When oxymetazoline and lidocaine are used together, pain due to endoscopy is reduced significantly [9].

The recommended dose of 0.05% oxymetazoline in adults and children over the age of 6 years is 2–3 sprays in each nostril not more than every 10–12 h. Oxymetazoline may increase mean blood pressure after its application, and this effect of oxymetazoline is not seen when it is combined with lidocaine [9]. There is always a suspicion that local decongestants may cause hypertension and reflex bradycardia [13], therefore, the physicians use decongestants carefully in elderly patients and in patients with cardiovascular diseases.

4.3.3 Anti-Secretion Medications

Nasal secretions and saliva can hinder the view from the fiberscope. Secretions dilute the local anesthetics, create a barrier between mucosa and local anesthetics; therefore, the absorption of local anesthetics are hindered. The anticholinergic agents are commonly used to address this problem [14].

The medication most commonly used is glycopyrrolate followed by atropine and scopolamine. Glycopyrrolate has several advantages including lack of central nervous system effects (it does not cross the blood brain barrier) and less tachycardia than atropine. A dose of 3–4 μg/kg is suggested, or for most adults 0.2 mg. If the IM route is chosen, it should be given at least 15 minutes before [15].

4.4 Procedures

4.4.1 Patient Preparation

Vocal fold injections are usually performed with the patient awake with cooperation. The physician explains the procedures to the patient and an informed consent is obtained. Cardiopulmonary monitoring is not usually performed before or during the procedure. Patients can be seated on an ENT chair or supine according to the injection procedure position.

Vocal fold injections are safe procedure and end usually quickly. Therefore, a peripheral intravenous (IV) line is not mandatory. The primary purpose of preparation of peripheral IV line is not for therapeutic purposes such as administration of medications, but for in emergency status such as anaphylactic shock or vasovagal syncope. Local anesthesia and manipulation of nasal cavity and oropharynx may cause a vasovagal response. If a sign or symptom of syncope occurs, including nausea, sweating, lightheadedness, and paresthesia, the procedure should be discontinued and the patient placed in a supine position [7].

4.4.2 Nasal Anesthesia

Nasal anesthesia is most commonly obtained by topical techniques. An infiltration (injection) of any anesthetics and direct nerve blocks are rarely necessary during vocal fold injection. The use of a decongestant spray before the topical anesthetic spray reduces its systemic absorption and reduces bleeding by laryngoscopy [7].

The patient's more patent nasal cavity is prepared. First, topical agents may be sprayed, followed by placement into the nasal cavity of cotton pledgets soaked in topical agents; lidocaine and oxymetazoline. Typically, three pledgets are placed in nasal cavity. The first pledget is placed horizontally on the floor of the nasal cavity and stacked each subsequent pledget on top of the first. Squeezing any excess anesthetic from the pledget is reducing excessive systemic absorption. The pledgets are removed after 5–10 min, just before procedure.

4.4.3 Pharyngeal Anesthesia

Pharyngeal anesthesia is delivered by simply spray. The oropharynx is sprayed with topical 10% xylocaine (AstraZeneca, Luton, UK) or 10% lidocaine (Beracaine spray, Firson, Chungcheonam-do, Korea) and the patient is asked to swallow immediately [16].

A low-flow nebulizer can be used. The patient should inhale nebulized 3 mL of lidocaine 4%. This method can anesthetize the larynx simultaneously, but it takes more time than spray technique and needs specific equipment, a nebulizer itself.

4.4.4 Laryngeal Anesthesia

There are numerous laryngeal anesthesia techniques, the following three methods are commonly used. The simplest way is the using of 10% lidocaine spray or 10% xylocaine spray. In this method, pharyngeal and laryngeal anesthesia can be delivered simultaneously. One or two times of spray (10 ~ 20 mg of lidocaine) is applied to the soft palate and the base of tongue for pharyngeal anesthesia. Under the guidance of rigid laryngoscope, two more sprays are applied to the vocal folds and the epiglottis when the patient phonates/e/, producing characteristic "laryngeal gargle." An Abraham laryngeal cannula can also be used. A 10 ml syringe of 4% lidocaine attached to an Abraham cannula is passed from the oral cavity into the pharynx under laryngoscopy guidance. Approximately 1 ml is dripped over the tongue base, and 2 ~ 4 ml are more dripped onto the vocal fold during laryngeal gargle.

Second method is the direct application of anesthetics via the fiber-optic scope channel when the scope is positioned directly above the larynx. Briefly, a channeled flexible distal chip laryngoscope is passed through the anesthetized nasal cavity along the floor of the nose and advanced into the oropharynx. 1-mL aliquots of 4% lidocaine are then applied to the patient's endolarynx through the working channel of the laryngoscope while the patient holds a long/e/. At the end of the phonatory gesture, patients are instructed to breathe in deeply to inspire the lidocaine solution into the trachea if it was necessary [16, 17].

A cotton ball soaked in lidocaine 4% can be used to apply the anesthesia; grasp the soaked cotton ball with laryngeal forceps, then, with the tongue grasped, apply the cotton ball transorally to the epiglottis, hypopharynx, and vocal fold mucosal surfaces. A thorough pharyngeal anesthesia should be done before this method for preventing gag reflex.

4.4.5 Skin Anesthesia

For percutaneous vocal fold injection (via transcricothyroid membrane or transthyrohyoid membrane), the area overlying the injection site should be anesthetized. To anesthetize the skin and subcutaneous tissues, a lidocaine 1% with epinephrine 1:100,000 or without epinephrine is most commonly used.

4.5 Medical Concerns

Patients must not be administered an anesthetic agent to which they are allergic. Use of internal swabs or pledgets soaked in vasoconstrictors is contraindicated in patients with uncontrolled hypertension or coronary artery disease [13]. There may be a significant change in heart rate during the procedure due to anxiety; furthermore, the placement of the scope in the nasopharynx and hypopharynx was associated with a significant rise in systolic blood pressure and heart rate, respectively.

While the amount of topical and local anesthetics used in injection laryngoplasty rarely exceeds toxic doses, the physician should be aware of the toxic dosages and the signs, symptoms, and treatment of anesthetic toxicity [18].

Topical anesthetic agents may cause discomfort/pain, burning/stinging sensation, gagging/nausea, unpleasant taste, globus sensation, dysphasia, or dyspnea [7, 9]. The anesthetic effect on the larynx and trachea may also result in a sensation that a patient cannot breathe [3]. Patients should be instructed to take nothing by mouth for approximately 60–90 min after the procedures to prevent aspiration.

Key Learning Points:

- Vocal fold injections are performed with the patient awake with cooperation. The physician explains the procedures to the patient and an informed consent is obtained.
- For comfortable and safe office-based procedures, thorough anesthesia should be provided to the following three regions; nasal cavity, oropharynx, and larynx.
- Lidocaine, tetracaine, prilocaine, ropivacaine, and bupivacaine have been used in the office-based procedures.
- Lidocaine has a low to intermediate potency, 45 to 60 minutes duration of action, and onset of sufficient anesthesia within 90 seconds of topical administration.
- Nasal decongestant, oxymetazoline, is used for widening nasal cavity by constriction of nasal mucosa.
- Cardiopulmonary monitoring is not usually performed before or during the procedure.
- The amount of topical anesthetics rarely exceeds toxic doses, it may cause some side effects; discomfort, burning sensation, nausea, and unpleasant taste, etc.

References

1. Ballard DP, Abramowitz J, Sukato DC, Bentsianov B, Rosenfeld RM. Systematic review of voice outcomes for injection Laryngoplasty performed under local vs general anesthesia. Otolaryngol - Head Neck Surg. 2018;159:608–14.
2. Frosh AC, Jayaraj S, Porter G, Almeyda J. Is local anaesthesia actually beneficial in flexible fibreoptic nasendoscopy? Clin Otolaryngol Allied Sci. 1998;23:259–62.
3. Gaviola GC, Chen V, Chia SH. A prospective, randomized, double-blind study comparing the efficacy of topical anesthetics in nasal endoscopy. Laryngoscope. 2013;123:852–8.
4. Cain AJ, Murray DP, McClymont LG. The use of topical nasal anaesthesia before flexible nasendoscopy: a double-blind, randomized controlled trial comparing cophenylcaine with placebo. Clin Otolaryngol Allied Sci. 2002;27:485–8.
5. Haytoğlu S, Kuran G, Muluk NB, Arıkan OK. Different anesthetic agents-soaked sinus packings on pain management after functional endoscopic sinus surgery: which is the most effective? Eur Arch Oto-Rhino-Laryngology. 2016;273:1769–77.
6. Hornung DE. Nasal anatomy and the sense of smell. Adv Otorhinolaryngol. 2006;63:1–22.
7. Wang SX, Simpson CB. Anesthesia for office procedures. Otolaryngol Clin N Am. 2013;46:13–9.
8. Yoshida Y, Tanaka Y, Hirano M, Nakashima T. Sensory innervation of the pharynx and larynx. Am J Med. 2000;108:51–61.
9. Şahin Mİ, Kökoğlu K, Güleç Ş, Ketenci İ, Ünlü Y. Premedication methods in nasal endoscopy: a prospective, randomized, double-blind study. Clin Exp Otorhinolaryngol. 2017;10:158–63.
10. Gencer ZK, Özkiriş M, Gencer M, Saydam L (2013) Comparison of ropivacaine, bupivacaine, prilocaine,andlidocaine in the management of pain and hemorrhage during nasal pack removal. Am J Rhinol Allergy 27:423–425.
11. Cherobin ACFP, Tavares GT. Safety of local anesthetics. An Bras Dermatol. 2020;95:82–90.
12. Bourolias C, Gkotsis A, Kontaxakis A, Tsoukarelis P. Lidocaine spray vs tetracaine solution for transnasal fiber-optic laryngoscopy. Am J Otolaryngol - Head Neck Med Surg. 2010;31:114–6.
13. Latham GJ, Jardine DS. Oxymetazoline and hypertensive crisis in a child: can we prevent it? Paediatr Anaesth. 2013;23:952–6.
14. Prasanna D, Bhat S. Nasotracheal intubation: an overview. J Maxillofac Oral Surg. 2014;13:366–72.
15. (2012) Awake Bronchoscopic Intubation. In: Univ. Heal. Netw.
16. McPartlin DW, Nouraei SAR, Tatla T, Howard DJ, Sandhu GS. How we do it: Transnasal fibreoptic oesophagoscopy. Clin Otolaryngol. 2005;30:547–50.
17. Verma SP, Smith ME, Dailey SH. Transnasal tracheoscopy. Laryngoscope. 2012;122:1326–30.
18. Neal JM, Bernards CM, Butterworth JF, Di Gregorio G, Drasner K, Hejtmanek MR, Mulroy MF, Rosenquist RW, Weinberg GL. ASRA practice advisory on local anesthetic systemic toxicity. Reg Anesth Pain Med. 2010;35:152–61.

Part II

Approaches for Vocal Fold Injection

5 Trans-Oral Approach

Pavan S. Mallur and Clark A. Rosen

Abstract

Trans-oral vocal fold injection is the only non-percutaneous approach for vocal fold augmentation routinely performed in awake patients. With this approach, the operator manipulates a curved needle from the oral cavity to the glottis, visualizing with assistant-driven flexible trans-nasal or surgeon-driven rigid peroral laryngoscopy. This is a technically challenging approach predicated on the coordinated abilities of the surgeon and assistant. Moreover, success is highly dependent on patient factors, as unfavorable anatomy or a strong oropharyngeal gag may preclude completion of the procedure. Despite this, the trans-oral approach provides excellent needle control allowing for high precision in directing needle placement and controlling the nature of vocal fold augmentation.

P. S. Mallur
Department of Otolaryngology Head and Neck Surgery, Harvard Medical School, Boston, MA, USA
e-mail: pmallur@bidmc.harvard.edu

C. A. Rosen (✉)
Division of Laryngology,
Department of Otolaryngology Head and Neck Surgery, UCSF Voice & Swallowing Center, University of California,
San Francisco, California, USA
e-mail: clark.rosen@ucsf.edu

Keywords

Deep vocal fold injection · Injection augmentation · Awake laryngeal procedures · Vocal fold paralysis · Vocal fold paresis · Vocal fold atrophy · Trial vocal fold injection

5.1 Introduction

The trans-oral approach to vocal fold injection was first described by Bruening in 1911 with the use of paraffin for vocal fold augmentation [1]. Since the initial description, advances in office laryngoscopy, instrumentation, and injection materials have made the trans-oral approach a fundamental technique for awake vocal fold injection [2, 3]. With this technique, a surgeon directs a curved needle through a patient's oral cavity, oropharynx, and supraglottis to the vocal folds; this critically involves an uninterrupted path caudal to the soft palate, cranial and then posterior to the epiglottis, and anterior to the arytenoid cartilages. Traditionally, an assistant simultaneously performs trans-nasal flexible laryngoscopy to provide visualization for the surgeon beyond the oropharynx [4]. Alternatively, the surgeon may perform both needle placement and visualization via trans-oral laryngoscopy with a 70- or 90-degree rigid telescope.

The trans-oral technique is the only awake technique for vocal fold augmentation that provides a direct transluminal pathway to the vocal fold. In contrast, the trans-cricothyroid and trans-

© Springer Nature Singapore Pte Ltd. 2021

B.-J. Lee et al. (eds.), *Vocal Fold Injection*, https://doi.org/10.1007/978-981-16-3303-4_5

thyroid cartilage approaches utilize blind percutaneous pathways and rely on transmitted submucosal motion of the needle tip to determine needle tip location. The thyrohyoid approach allows for endoluminal needle tip visualization however utilizes a percutaneous pathway as well [5]. Finally, injection augmentation via flexible needle through a channel laryngoscope has been described, though in clinical practice is not utilized widely [6].

There are a number of advantages the trans-oral approach has over the other described techniques. The principle advantage is the high degree of control achieved with direct needle manipulation and visualization which allows for directed needle placement along one or multiple punctum and with accurate control of depth of insertion. This avoids the dangers inherit in the blind percutaneous pathways and allows for robust control of augmentation and even focal vocal fold augmentation. The control and precision of needle placement and vocal fold augmentation is primal to achieve consistent, high-quality vocal fold augmentation results. As part of the procedure, direct palpation of the vocal process can be achieved to diagnose neurogenic paralysis/paresis versus cricoarytenoid joint fixation. Similarly, vocal fold free edge palpation can be performed to assess for focal lamina deficits, pathology, and scar.

The disadvantages of the approach arise from both technical nuances and patient factors. The approach is technically challenging with a steep learning curve that may be difficult to master without formal training and adequate volume. An additional challenge arises with assistant-driven visualization, as an experienced endoscopist is needed to simultaneously provide visualization of the needle and vocal folds without physically impeding the needle trajectory [4]. Stepwise coordination requires an experienced team. Specific to patient anatomy, airway crowding may make visualization or access more difficult; prominent base of tongue, retroflexed epiglottis, pharyngeal wall crowding, and overhanging arytenoid cartilages are all potential anatomical limitations., Finally, strong oropharyngeal gag is most commonly the limiting factor preventing trans-oral access and completion of the injection.

5.2 Indications for Trans-Oral Technique

Indications for the trans-oral approach include the need for temporary or durable augmentation for mild-to-moderate glottic insufficiency associated with vocal fold immobility / paralysis, hypomobility/paresis, atrophy, and other select cases of glottic insufficiency. The precision of the trans-oral approach make it especially useful for focal augmentation; this may arise with global atrophy requiring mid-membranous augmentation, post-surgical soft tissue deficit, and focal glottic insufficiency due to scar. The trans-oral approach may be preferred over percutaneous approach in patients with difficult neck anatomy where normal landmarks are not readily palpable; this may be found in patients with previous neck surgery, head and neck cancer or other soft tissue masses, obese patients, or severe kyphosis or scoliosis of the cervical spine. Finally, the trans-oral approach can be used to confirm presence or absence of vocal fold fixation/arytenoid joint dislocation by allowing palpation of the arytenoid and vocal process.

5.3 Contraindications for Trans-Oral Technique

There are several relative contraindications to attempting the trans-oral technique for vocal fold injection. The most commonly encountered is a hyperactive orpharyngeal gag; while it is possible to suppress this with topical anesthesia and/or intravenous sedation, in some cases it cannot be overcome which makes an alternative approach necessary [7]. Similarly crowded pharyngeal anatomy, overhanging arytenoid cartilage and mucosa, and large cervical spine osteophytes, or significant trismus may preclude successful trans-oral approach. Patients that cannot remain seated upright or relatively still and patients with limited limb mobility are also suboptimal candidates, as sniffing position and the patient holding their own tongue facilitates this approach. Active anticoagulation or antiplatelet therapy is not a firm contraindication as intraluminal hemorrhage causing airway compromise is exceedingly rare [8]. Comparing the bleeding risk of a trans-oral approach versus the percutaneous approaches has not been done, the former involves mucosal violation but the latter involves passing the needle through deep laryngeal tissues. Finally, the trans-oral needle is typically a 22- to 25-cm-long 16 g shaft ending in a 24 g or 27 g needle. Considering these parameters and viscosity of injection materials, it is not surprising that injection takes considerable pressure and a threshold level of hand strength to achieve.

5.4 Anesthesia

Local anesthesia is typically sufficient for completion of the trans-oral injection. Nasal anesthesia and decongestants are applied with nasal pledgets or cottinoids soaked with a 1:1 mixture of 4% lidocaine and oxymetazoline or neosynephrine. A nebulization of 4–5 cm^3 of 4% lidocaine run with 4 L of oxygen provides global anesthesia of the oropharynx, larynx and subglottic airway. Focal anesthesia is achieved via a drip catheter through the channel laryngoscope; single droplets of 4% lidocaine are placed along the base of tongue and laryngeal surface of the epiglottis. Following this step, the patient is asked to phonate while 0.25–0.5 cm^3 of 4% lidocaine is placed onto the false vocal fold and asked to cough following phonation; the phonation provides anesthesia directly to the vocal folds while phonation and cough distributes the lidocaine throughout the laryngopharynx and prevents transtracheal absorption of lidocaine. Efficacy of topicalization can be assessed by using the drip catheter to directly apply 1–2 drops of 4% lidocaine onto the vocal fold followed by direct palpation with the catheter. Following this, topical benzocaine or lidocaine spray can be applied peroral to the soft palate and posterior pharyngeal wall if needed. At this point, the anesthesia level can be tested by simulating the injection trajectory using a blunt tip curved cannula such as the Abraham Laryngeal Cannula (Becton-Dickinson, Teleflex). Other similar commercially available cannula includes the Joussen Larynx Cannula (Karl Storz), Laryngeal Cannula (BR Surgical), and Andrew-Pynchon Suction Tube (Jarit).

Select circumstances may warrant administration of conscious sedation or anxiolytics to help facilitate patient tolerance and completion of the procedure. In the inpatient or hospital setting, trans-oral injection may be performed in a procedural or operating suite; intravenous midazolam or remifentanil with or without dexmedetomidine may be administered with appropriate cardiopulmonary monitoring. In the outpatient or ambulatory setting, a cooperative but anxious patient may benefit from an oral benzodiazepine taken several hours prior to the procedure; diazepam 1 mg or alprazolam 0.25–0.5 mg is typically sufficient to serve as an anxiolytic without excessive sedation in the benzodiazepine naïve patient.

5.5 Equipment and Injection Material

The equipment required for trans-oral injection centers around need for visualization and administration of topical anesthesia. Laryngoscopy tower capable of transmitting digital laryngoscopy across 1–2 monitors provides a central point of visualization for the surgeon and assistant. Targeted topicalization of 4% lidocaine to the laryngopharynx is best achieved via a spray catheter directed through a laryngoscope with working channel. The channel laryngoscope additionally has suction capability for secretion management. If channel laryngoscopes are not available, directing a red-rubber catheter through the opposite nasal cavity has been described for the laryngeal gargle. A malleable blunt tip catheter with Luer lock adaptor, most commonly the Abraham laryngeal cannula, may serve several functions in the procedure; this may be used to delivery topical lidocaine to the base of tongue and endolarynx, allow for palpation of the arytenoid/vocal process, help estimate the needle trajectory required for injection, and allow the injector and assistant to coordinate their actions.

There are numerous commercially available injection materials with variable duration of efficacies. These include carboxymethyl cellulose (Prolaryn™ Gel, Renu® Gel), hyaluronic acid (Restylane®) or cross-linked hyaluronic acid (Juvederm®), and calcium hydroxylapatite (Prolaryn™ Voice, Renu® Voice). A malleable 24 g trans-oral needle with Luer lock is packaged with Prolaryn™ injectables, and available separately with Renu® injectables. Alternatively, reusable trans-oral injection cannula with disposable needles are available, such as the Integra® Life Sciences curved laryngeal injection cannula; because these only allow for 1 cm^3 tuberculin syringes and use 27 g needles, they are optimally used for Botox, superficial steroid, and subepithelial saline injection.

5.6 Procedure

5.6.1 Setup and Positioning

During the trans-oral approach, the patient is seated up right with slight flexion at the waist and neck and slight head extension to facilitate visual and instrument access to the larynx. Additionally, the patient is asked to use the left hand to manually retract the tongue anteriorly, opening up the oropharyngeal and supraglottic space. The right-handed surgeon will typically stand to the right and slightly anterior to the patient, with the assistant driving the flexible laryngoscope standing on the left and slightly anterior to the patient. Laryngoscopy tower and primary monitor is typically placed behind and to the left of the patient; to this end, a monitor mounted on an articulating arm helps optimize monitor placement to the surgeon and assistant's line of view. Alternatively, a second monitor may be placed to the right and posterior to the patient directly across the assistant driving the flexible laryngoscope. Injection materials and other equipment may be kept in front and to the left of the surgeon on a small Mayo stand. An additional assistant to hand the surgeon instruments directly is helpful, but not necessary (Fig. 5.1).

5.6.2 Trajectory Approximation and Arytenoid Palpation

Use of a malleable blunt tip cannula, such as the Abraham laryngeal cannula is an important step that serves four distinct purposes; the surgeon is able to (1) assess patient tolerance, (2) estimate trajectory needed for injection, (3) palpate the arytenoid cartilage/vocal process to rule out mechanical fixation of an immobile vocal fold, and (4) coordinate planned movement with the assistant driving the laryngoscope. Following all steps of topical anesthesia, the assistant maintains the flexible laryngoscope in the oropharynx, while the patient grasps the tongue for anterior retraction. The surgeon uses a tongue depressor for the oral tongue, and maintains the curved cannula in a horizontal position through the oropharynx. Once past the soft palate, the surgeon rotates the cannula counterclockwise while simultaneously advancing the cannula tip past the epiglottis. As a safety check, this allows patients with a strong oropharyngeal gag to declare themselves with a blunt instrument in place rather than a sharp needle point. Typically, the angle of trajectory from oropharynx to posterior one-third of the membranous vocal fold is 90-degrees; the exact angle and more variable distance can be estimated using the malleable Abraham cannula. Finally, the cannula can be used to place gentle lateral pressure on the vocal process or medial surface of the arytenoid; this allows surgeon to evaluate an immobile vocal fold for fixation by directly viewing passing mobility with palpation (Fig. 5.2a).

5.6.3 Technique

The trans-oral approach with the needle will replicate the trial with Abraham cannula, with the assistant initially maintaining the flexible

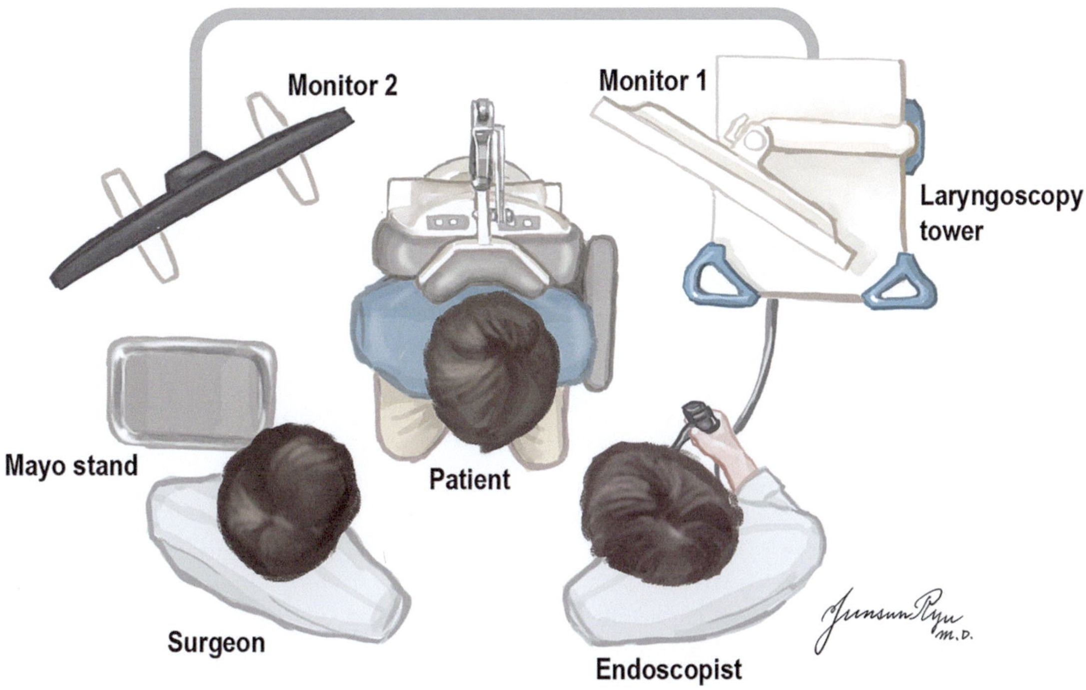

Fig. 5.1 (Redrawn based on Mallur PS and Rosen CA. Office-Based Laryngeal Injections. *Otolaryngol Clin N Am* 2013; 46: 85–100). Spatial orientation of surgeon, assistant, patient, and equipment during transoral vocal fold injection

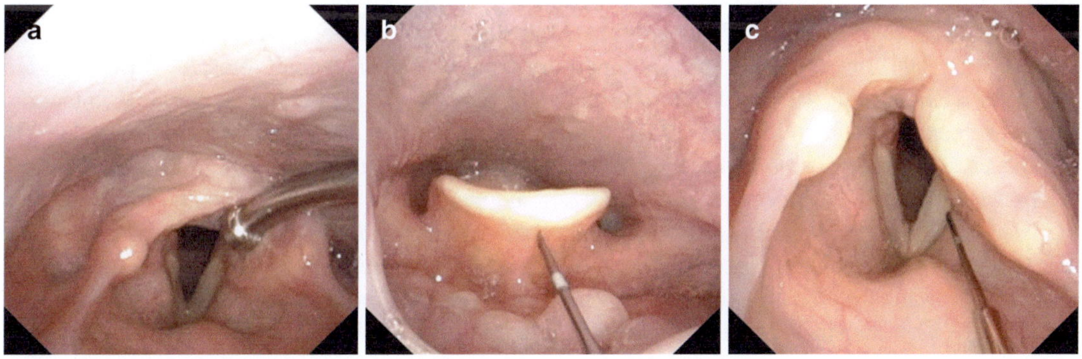

Fig. 5.2 (**a**). Palpation of vocal process/arytenoid with blunt tip cannula, demonstrating passive abduction and absence of fixation. (**b**). Visualization of the needle point past the soft palate via flexible laryngoscopy. (**c**). Typical trajectory of needle toward insertion point (marked X) lateral to TA muscle in posterior one-third of membranous vocal fold

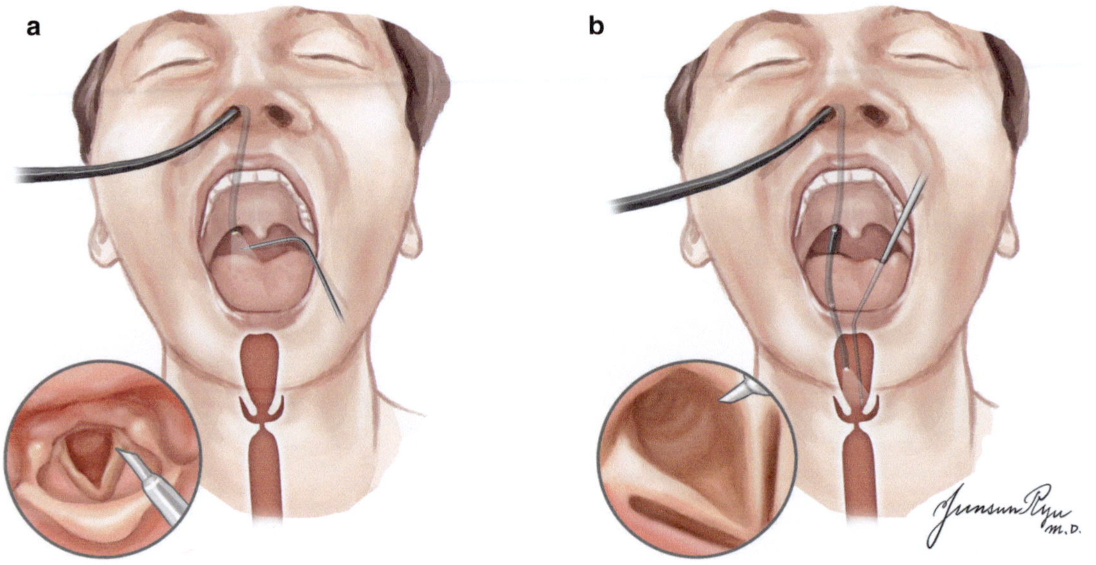

Fig. 5.3 (Redrawn based on Mallur PS and Rosen CA. Techniques for the Laryngology Assistant: Providing Optimal Visualization. *Oper Techniques Otolaryngol* 2012; 25:197–202). Needle trajectory during transoral vocal fold injection. (**a**). Horizontal entry of needle into oropharynx with laryngoscope at the soft palate level. (**b**). Advancement of laryngoscope opposite to needle and vocal fold to be injected

laryngoscope at the soft palate level and the surgeon introducing the needle horizontally into the oropharynx (Fig. 5.3a). It is sometimes helpful to utilize the nasal cavity opposite the vocal fold to be injected. The surgeon may use a tongue depressor initially until the needle tip is visualized on screen, after which the tongue depressor is removed (Fig. 5.2b). Using the left hand within the oral cavity to guide trajectory and stabilize the needle, the surgeon advances the needle forward while rotating counter-clockwise with the right hand toward the vocal fold to be injected (Fig. 5.2c). The assistant should advance the laryngoscope to the side opposite of the vocal fold to be injected; if the left vocal fold is to be injected, the laryngoscope should remain to the right of the needle and vice versa for the opposite vocal fold. This prevents direct interference with the needle and allows for an unobstructed view of the vocal fold superior surface, free edge, and infraglottis (Fig. 5.3b). This visualization is essential to the success of high quality, detailed vocal fold augmentation

The initial target for needle insertion should be posterior membranous vocal fold, just lateral to the thyroarytenoid muscle. Insertion too medial risks subepithelial/superficial injection, while insertion too lateral into the ventricle risks a paraglottic injection with limited vocal fold augmentation. Once insertion is complete to a depth of approximately 5 mm, the assistant should advance the laryngoscope to allow for a view of the free edge and infraglottic aspect of the vocal fold. A small volume of material can be injected as a test to ensure there is no subepithelial injection or egress into the infraglottic/subglottic lumen. Augmentation should proceed at this point, with infraglottic augmentation typically preceding the glottic level augmentation. If there is excessive infraglottic augmentation, the needle can be withdrawn slightly; care must be taken with this step, as it can result in superficial injection into the Reinke's space. If additional, or focal augmentation is needed, the needle is withdrawn and reinserted lateral to the thyroarytenoid muscle where augmentation is needed. Following injection of one vocal fold, the assistant withdraws the laryngoscope to the soft palate level and the surgeon withdraws the needle and directs it toward the opposite vocal fold by simultaneously moving the entire needle complex contralaterally toward the opposite vocal fold. Similarly, the assistant advances the laryngoscope opposite the vocal fold to be injected. At several time points during the procedure, the surgeon can assess the result of the augmentation by evaluating the voice quality, vocal fold closure, and vocal fold vibration via stroboscopy.

An alternative trans-oral approach utilizes surgeon-provided visualization with a rigid telescope. A right-handed surgeon will hold a 70° or 90° telescope coupled to a camera head in the left hand, and the needle in the right hand. The patient protrudes then grasps his or her own tongue with a dry gauze. The surgeon will visualize the larynx with the telescope while the needle is introduced peroral and advanced past the oropharynx toward the vocal fold. The surgeon may choose to angle the telescope for optimal visualization, and injection proceeds as described above.

5.6.4 Complications

Complications encountered with trans-oral approach to vocal fold injection are fortunately rare and often self-limiting. The most common complication encountered is inability to tolerate trans-oral injection to completion; this may be due to copious secretions, strong oropharyngeal gag or cough, or more rarely difficult anatomy such as retroflexed epiglottis or overhanging arytenoid cartilage [7].

With actual mucosal penetration, bleeding may occur either intraluminally or within the paraglottic space due to a small vessel. With intraluminal bleeding, the patient should be observed with the flexible laryngoscope in place until no active bleeding is seen. Readministration of topical lidocaine and suctioning of excess blood can help prevent reactive laryngospasm and cough. Failing control, the patient should be taken to an appropriate setting for general anesthesia, direct laryngoscopy, and direct compression with 1:10,000 epinepherine soaked pledgets. Paraglottic hemorrhage can be identified with rapidly developing medialization and edema of the vocal folds following injection. It is often self-limited to the physical constraints of the paraglottic space, however repeated visualization for airway compromise should be performed 30 min following cessation. With bilateral paraglottic hemorrhage, an oral corticosteroid taper is often warranted, and a minority of patients may benefit from intravenous corticosteroids and inpatient observation for airway compromise.

Superficial injection into Reinke's space is another complication that may occur with a trans-oral approach. This can also occur with the trans-cricothyroid or trans-thyroid cartilage approaches. This can be identified readily with hydrodissection of the subepithelial space and lifting of the epithelium that is distinct from augmentation seen with deep injection. This disrupts the normal rheologic properties of the superficial lamina propria, resulting in significant dysphonia with a high-pitch and harsh quality. With carboxymethyl cellulose, hyaluronic acid, and collagen, superficial injection can be managed expectantly for resolution which may take up to several weeks or months. Superficial calcium hydroxylapetite injection carries risk for significant inflammatory reaction with scar formation and should prompt attempts at removal [9]. In an awake patient, the Abraham catheter may be used to manually express material from the injection punctum; this can be better achieved by making a 1–2 mm incision at the injection site with the injection needle. If immediate removal of superficial injection is not possible, removal of the calcium hydroxylapetite under microlaryngoscopy should be planned within several days.

5.6.5 Post-Injection

Following an uncomplicated trans-oral approach to vocal fold injection, the patient is usually observed clinically without laryngoscopy for 15 min. The patient should remain NPO for at least 60 min to prevent aspiration until the effects of topical anesthesia dissipate. Voice rest for 24 h is sometimes recommended for two reasons; this may prevent material extrusion while the needle puncture site seals and may prevent development of subepithelial hemorrhage. Patients usually do not need systemic oral analgesics though short burst of oral corticosteroids can help any developing edema and expedite return to normal voicing.

Key Learning Points:

- Trans-oral injection is one of several ways to perform awake vocal fold injection augmentation for glottic insufficiency.
- The technique utilizes a curved needle directed peroral to the vocal fold with visualization via flexible laryngoscopy.
- The technique requires appropriate patient selection for absence of hyperactive gag and cough, favorable pharyngeal and supraglottic anatomy, ability of patient to remain upright for 1 h.
- The approach is technically challenging with a steep learning curve.
- The approach requires a skilled endoscopist to coordinate visualization with the surgeon.
- The technique provides the surgeon the most control of needle placement and best chance for precision vocal fold injection.
- Is particularly useful when precise and focal augmentation is needed for atrophy and focal glottic insufficiency, such as soft tissue deficit, sulcus vocalis, and scar.

References

1. Bruening W. Uber eine neue Behandlungsmethode der Rekurrenslamung [in German]. Verh Verl Deutsch Laryngol. 1911;18:93–151.
2. Courey MS. Injection laryngoplasty. Otolaryngol Clin N Am. 2004;37:121–38.
3. Sulica L, Rosen CA, Postma GN, Simpson B, Amin M, et al. Current practice in injection augmentation of the vocal folds: indications, treatment principles, techniques, and complications. Laryngoscope. 2010;120(2):319–25.
4. Mallur PS, Rosen CA. Techniques for the laryngology assistant: providing optimal visualization. Op Tech Otolaryngol. 2012;23(3):197–202.
5. Amin MA. Thyrohyoid approach for vocal fold augmentation. Ann Otol Rhinol Laryngol. 2006;115(9):699–702.
6. Trask DK, Shellenberger DL, Hoffman HT. Transnasal, endoscopic vocal fold augmentation. Laryngoscope. 2005;115(12):2262–5.
7. Young VN, Smith LJ, Sulica L, Krishna PK, Rosen CA. Patient tolerance of awake, in-office laryngeal procedures: a multi-institutional perspective. Laryngoscope. 2010;122(2):315–21.
8. Fritz MA, Peng R, Born H, Cerrati EW, Verma A, Wang B, Branski RC, Amin MR. The safety of antithrombotic therapy during in-office laryngeal procedures: a preliminary study. J Voice. 2015;29(6): 768–71.
9. Chheda NN, Rosen CA, Belafsky PC, Simpson CB, Postma GN. Revision laryngeal surgery for the suboptimal injection of calcium hydroxylapatite. Laryngoscope. 2008;118(12):2260–3.

6 Trans-Cricothyroid Approach

Tack-Kyun Kwon

Abstract

Transcutaneous trans-cricothyroid (CT) vocal fold injection offers several advantages over any other approaches due to its short delivery route without crossing endolaryngeal mucosa, but also has a critical disadvantage coming from the invisible nature of the procedure. To overcome this disadvantage, surgeons should be familiar with the various techniques for identifying the exact level of the true vocal fold and estimating the exact location of the needle tip. Identification of inferior border of the thyroid cartilage is the most critical step to locate the level of the true vocal fold, and careful palpation with the needle within the vocal fold is the key to precise injection depth control. After the initial learning curve, trans-CT approach can be a safe, fast and simple option for vocal fold injection.

Keywords

Vocal fold injection · Injection laryngoplasty
Trans-cricothyroid approach · Transcutaneous injection

T.-K. Kwon (✉)
Department of Otorhinolaryngology-Head and Neck Surgery, Seoul National University College of Medicine, Seoul, South Korea
e-mail: kwontk@snu.ac.kr

6.1 Introduction

Vocal fold injection includes all procedures that deliver foreign materials into the vocal folds regardless of the injectable materials utilized. Injection laryngoplasty refers to the procedure that modifies the shape of the larynx by vocal fold injection.

The trans-CT approach was first reported in 1916 by Seifert, in which the needle enters the subglottic airway through CT membrane and is directed to the vocal fold [1]. A extramucosal trans-CT approach was introduced in 1985 by Ward et al. [2] and trans-nasal flexible laryngoscopy guided trans-CT approach was first described in 1990 by Hirano [3].

Trans-CT approach offers several advantages compared to other approaches [4, 5]:

1. Shorter delivery route makes easier to control the needle tip direction and the amount of injection.
2. No requirement for endolaryngeal anesthesia due to extramucosal needle passage.
3. Thicker soft tissue layers prevent backflow of the injection material.
4. Fast procedure while providing comfort to the patients (less pain and gag reflex).
5. No airway bleeding or spasm.

© Springer Nature Singapore Pte Ltd. 2021
B.-J. Lee et al. (eds.), *Vocal Fold Injection*, https://doi.org/10.1007/978-981-16-3303-4_6

However, this approach has also several disadvantages [6–8]:

1. The surgeon cannot see the needle tip, which means practically blinded procedure.
2. This approach necessitates an initial learning curve.

In this chapter, the author will describe detailed procedural steps of vocal fold injection via trans-CT approach and introduce various techniques for achieving successful results.

6.2 Surgical Techniques

6.2.1 Basic Steps for Vocal Fold Injection with Trans-CT Approach

The first and most crucial step in trans-CT injection is to identify the exact location of surgical landmarks. Especially in trans-CT approach, identification of the inferior border of the thyroid cartilage. After marking with surgical pen on the neck skin, the following steps are taken to prepare for the procedure:

First, the nose and pharynx are topically anesthetized with 4% lidocaine spray. A nasal decongestant can be applied if necessary. Because the most painful area for the patient during flexible laryngoscopy is the posterior aspect of nasal septum, posterior nasal packing with 1:1000 epinephrine and 2% lidocaine mixture can be a preferable alternative for nasal anesthesia. Hypopharyngeal or laryngeal anesthetic is not required for this approach because the needle does not touch the endolaryngeal mucosa. If the patient has a strong gag reflex, a few puffs of 4% topical lidocaine can be sprayed over the oropharynx. It is important not to spray too much because the injection procedure can become difficult due to increased airway secretion, aspiration, and cough reflex once the laryngeal mucosa is anesthetized.

Second, the surgical filed is disinfected with povidone-iodine or ethanol.

Then the skin around the CT membrane is infiltrated with 2% lidocaine. If the injection procedure is planned on the unilateral vocal fold, lidocaine infiltration is applied on the same side. Lidocaine infiltration covers from the skin to the cricothyroid membrane to reduce the patient's discomfort.The patient is seated comfortably on the unit chair, and allowed to lean backward and extend his or her neck for better exposure of the larynx during endoscopy. The endoscopist stands at the side of the chair according to his or her handedness. To avoid interference with the surgeon, the endoscopist can stand caudal to the patient. The endoscopist should have experience at managing the flexible laryngoscope so that the endoscope can be properly handled according to the patient's movement to avoid injury and the lens of the endoscope can easily be cleaned during the procedure.

The surgeon can sit or stand on the patient's side or caudal, depending on the surgeon's inclination. If the surgeon stands on one side of the patient, the endoscopist should stand on the other side of the patient even if the endoscope control might be more difficult due to his or her handedness (Fig. 6.1a).

If the surgeon stands on the top of the patient, he or she can utilize both hands and fingers more freely. Similar to anterior neck palpation during physical examination, multiple finger palpation is a more precise and sensitive way to identify surgical landmarks and locate the needle tip. Furthermore, the endoscopist and surgeon does not interfere with one another in this manner, and the endoscopist can have more room for the endoscope control regardless of the handedness. However, in this case, each endoscopist and surgeon should utilize two different monitors, one of which should be turned upside down because the vision is inverted (Fig. 6.1b).

Twenty-five gauge, 1.5-inch needle is most commonly used for trans-CT vocal fold injection. The needle should be primed with a small amount of injection material prior to the procedure. No warming of the syringe is required for highly viscous material because of the short injection route compared to transoral injection.

Before beginning the injection process, surgeons must first identify the exact location of the lower margin of the thyroid cartilage. In most

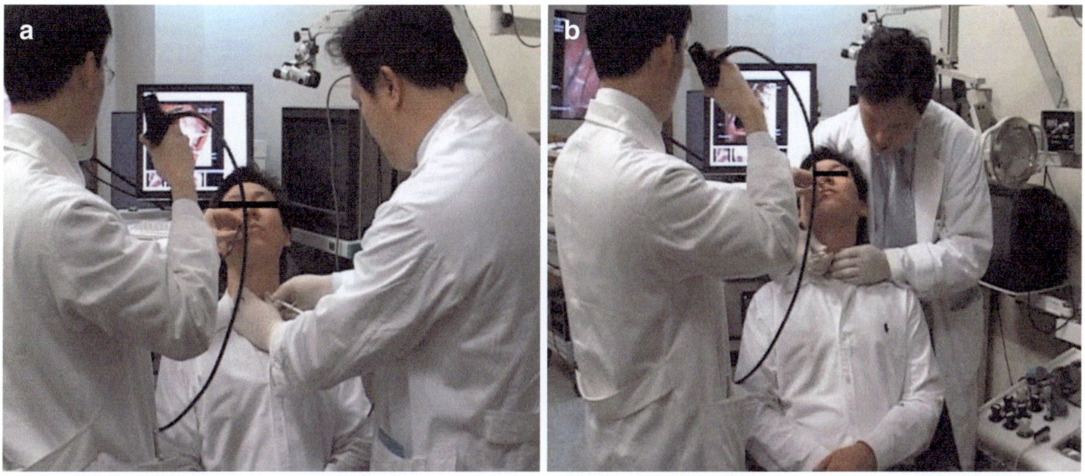

Fig. 6.1 The staffs position for the vocal fold injection. (**a**). The surgeon can sit or stand on one side of the patient while the endoscopist is on the other side. (**b**). The surgeon can stand on the top side of the patient while the endoscopist may stand on either side according to the handedness

cases, careful palpation with non-injecting hands is enough to identify cricothyroid space. The needle is inserted at the level of the lower border of the thyroid cartilage off the midline about 10–15 mm. The needle is then advanced steadily until the needle passes through the cricothyroid membrane. When the needle passes through the membrane, you may feel a small popping sense similar to that of poking a hole through a thin paper with a needle. If the needle passes through the cricothyroid membrane along the inferior border of the thyroid cartilage, the needle will readily enter the thyroarytenoid muscle in the infraglottic area. As the tip of the needle passes the cricothyroid membrane, the direction of the needle should be adjusted upward and lateral so that the tip of the needle can direct upward to the vocal fold at glottis level. If necessary, the needle can be slightly bent before the injection procedure. During the needle insertion procedure, the index finger of non-injecting hand should be placed on the cricothyroid space to guide the needle (Fig. 6.2).

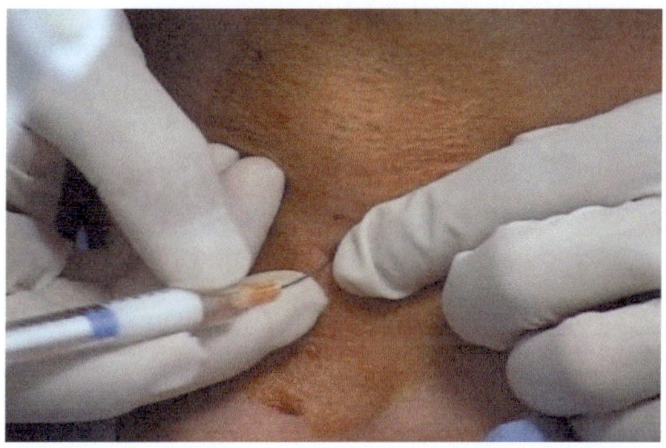

Fig. 6.2 The needle insertion with the finger palpation. Needle is inserted 5–10 mm off the midline while the location of the inferior border of the thyroid cartilage is continuously identified by the non-injecting hand

Once the needle enters the thyroarytenoid muscle, you can estimate the position and the depth of the needle tip by observing vocal fold movement from the endoscopic image on the monitor. The needle tip is progressively advanced to the location you wish to deliver the injection material while monitoring the direction and depth of the needle. After confirming the right position and depth of needle tip, you can start injecting by pushing the plunger with the non-injecting hand. At this point, you should anchor your injecting hand to the patient's neck with fingers to maintain the position of the needle tip. The plunger should be pushed gently and slowly to avoid abrupt injection of large amount or injection to the wrong place. By evaluating the vocal fold inflation, the surgeon can manage the amount of injection. In general, 10 ~ 20% over injection is suggested to be ideal in the literature, although there is no exact definition of over injection and no agreement of the appropriate injection volume.

6.2.2 Techniques to Locate the Level of the True Vocal Fold

The major downside of the trans-CT approach is the invisible needle tip during the procedure. To overcome this disadvantage, we need to practice various effective techniques to estimate precise location of the needle tip.

Jin et al. has reported the average angle and depth of the needle for trans-CT injection laryngoplasty for successful injection [9]. According to the findings, the distance from the skin to the posterior one-third area of the true vocal fold is 15.75 mm in men and 13.91 mm in women, and the angle needed to reach the target in the medial direction was 10.57° in men and 12.71° in women, and the angle needed in the superior direction was 47.57° in men and 47.43° in women. However, considering that the measurement is impractical during the procedure and that there are individual anatomical variances, more practical suggestion is required.

The cricothyroid space is clearly perceptible with fingers in most patients, and the inferior border of the thyroid cartilage is easily discernible merely by palpation, especially in slender patients. But in patient with obesity, previous history of neck surgery or radiation, those landmarks are difficult to identify with hands. In these cases, you can utilize one of following techniques.

1. Endoscopic observation with palpation: While observing anterior subglottis endoscopically, palpation of the neck with fingers helps you identify the cricothyroid space. Unless the anterior neck skin is substantially fibrosed, the cricothyroid space can be observed pushed back into the airway since it has no cartilaginous cover. Using this technique, you can estimate the level of the needle insertion while also identifying the midline (Fig. 6.3).
2. Endoscopic observation with needle probing: If the skin above the cricothyroid space is severely thick or hardened, the finger palpation may not reveal any changes. In this case, you can utilize the needle as a probe instead of using your fingertips. You should avoid puncturing the airway mucosa, since this can cause a cough reflex, airway bleeding and blurred vision due to bleeding (Fig. 6.4).

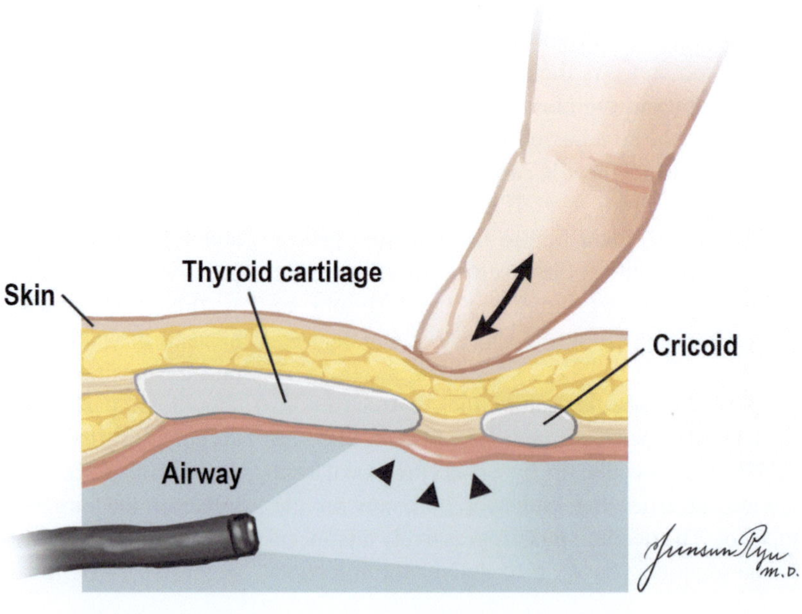

Fig. 6.3 Endoscopic identification of the vertical location of CT* membrane with finger palpation. With flexible laryngoscopic guidance, the level of the CT membrane can be determined by observing the mucosal elevation caused by the finger palpation over the CT membrane. **CT* cricothyroid

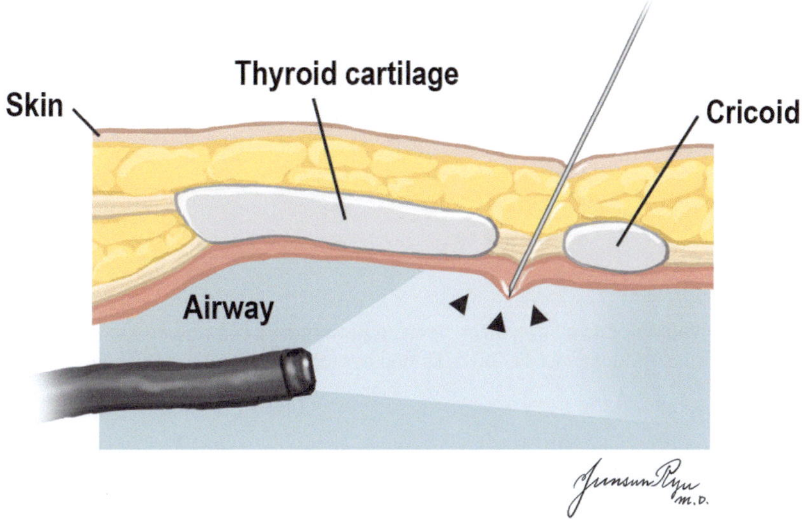

Fig. 6.4 Endoscopic identification of the vertical location of CT membrane with needle palpation. If the landmarks are difficult to locate, a needle palpation can be used instead of finger. Care should be taken not to penetrate the needle through the airway mucosa

3. Walking down technique: This technique is beneficial to all the patients regardless of their skin condition. First, insert the needle at the approximate vertical level of the inferior border of the thyroid cartilage 10–15 mm off the midline and advance deep until the thyroid cartilage is palpated with the needle tip. Then draw back the needle slightly, remaining in the subcutaneous space, and move the needle tip a little lower and palpate the cartilage again (Fig. 6.5a–d). This maneuver is repeated until the needle can slide in deeper without encountering the cartilaginous structure (Fig. 6.5e). Using this technique, you can insert the needle along the inferior border of the thyroid cartilage and enter the infraglottic level of the true vocal fold. At this point, change the direction of the needle upward and laterally, so the needle tip is placed in the thyroarytenoid muscle space.

6.2.3 Techniques to Estimate Exact Location of the Needle Tip

Once the needle tip enters the vocal fold, the free edge of the vocal fold will be observed to shift medially when you swing the syringe horizontally. By observing the vocal fold movement, you can approximate the longitudinal position of the needle tip (Fig. 6.6a). If you swing the syringe vertically, the vocal fold moves up and down, revealing the vertical location of the needle tip (Fig. 6.6b).

If the vocal fold is sharply lifted by the needle palpation, the needle is located in subepithelial space (Fig. 6.7a), so you should not inject filler agent in this region unless otherwise indicated. When you try to inject drugs into the subepithelial space, such as steroid or antiviral agents, this finding suggests the needle is in the appropriate space. If the vocal fold is bluntly elevated, the needle is located in subligamental space and ready for injection with filler material (Fig. 6.7b). If the whole length of vocal fold shifts medially, the needle is located lateral to the vocal process which is a suitable site for vocal fold augmentation of paralyzed vocal fold in far lateral position (Fig. 6.7c).

Many novel ideas have been reported in the literature to estimate the location of the needle tip during trans-CT approach. An EMG guided injection is one effort to overcome the blindness of trans-cricothyoid approach [10, 11]. The EMG indicates that the tip of the needle is positioned in the muscle, but it does not indicate the depth or longitudinal position of the needle in the thyroarytenoid muscle. Therefore this method should

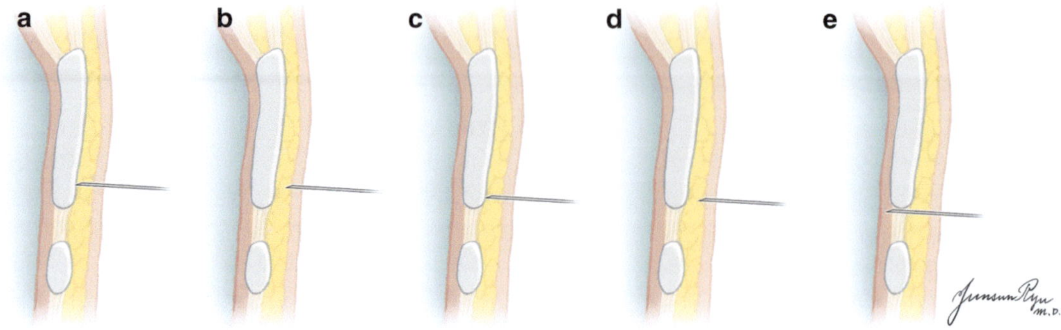

Fig. 6.5 "Walking down" technique. The inferior border of the thyroid cartilage is easily identified by probing the thyroid cartilage with the needle lowering step by step (**a**–**d**) until there is no palpable cartilage (**e**)

be employed for specific indications such as botulinum toxin injection or temporary vocal fold augmentation when a flexible endoscopy facility is not accessible.

Recently, Hoffman et al. developed transilluminated needle tip guided approach for real time light-guided cricothyroid approach [8] and Cha et al. improved technical issues using laser-guided needle [5]. By using a specially designed injection needle with optic fiber whithin, the operator can detect the location of the needle tip through endoscopic viewing of transillumination during the procedure (Fig. 6.8). The limitations of light-guided approach are the need for a larger bore needle for the optic fiber, and the invisibility of the needle tip after injecting opaque material.

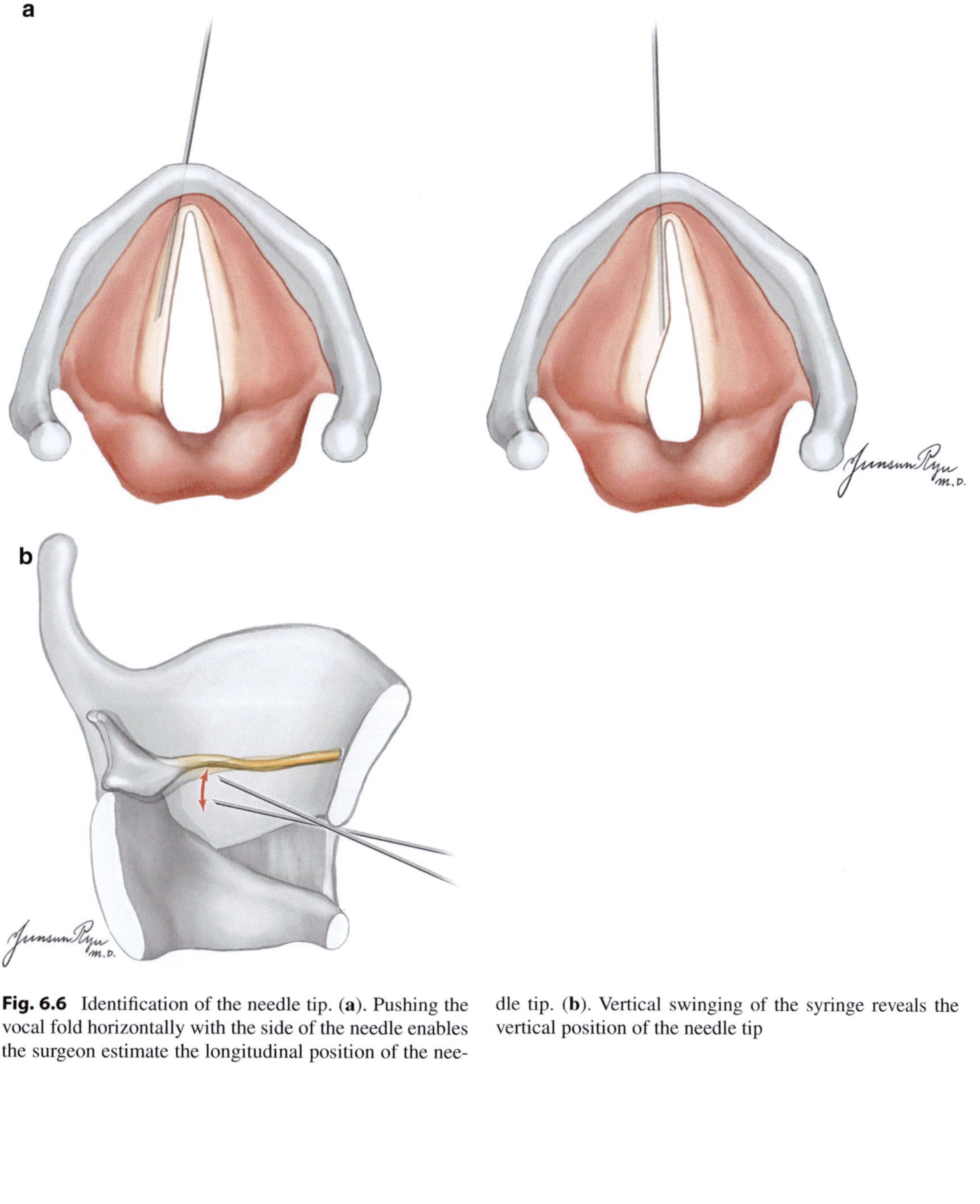

Fig. 6.6 Identification of the needle tip. (**a**). Pushing the vocal fold horizontally with the side of the needle enables the surgeon estimate the longitudinal position of the needle tip. (**b**). Vertical swinging of the syringe reveals the vertical position of the needle tip

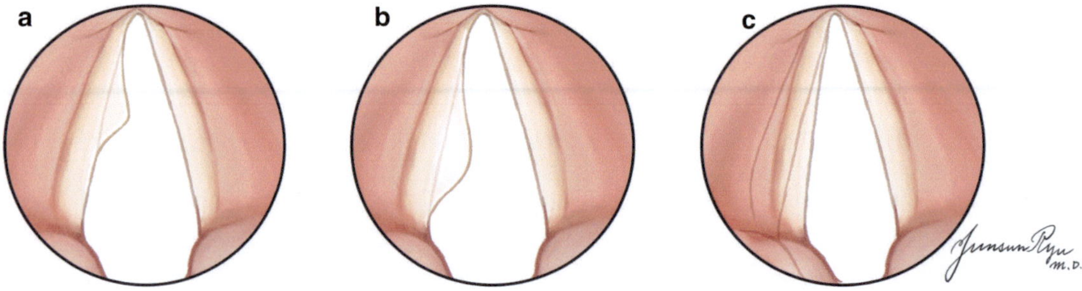

Fig. 6.7 Estimation of the needle depth according to the patterns of the vocal fold change during the needle palpation. (**a**). A sharp elevation of the vocal fold with the palpation indicates the needle is in the lamina propria space. (**b**). A blunt elevation of the vocal fold shows the needle location is deeper than the vocal ligament. (**c**). Medial displacement of the whole vocal fold on palpation indicates the needle tip is positioned in the lateral aspect of the vocal process of the arytenoid cartilage

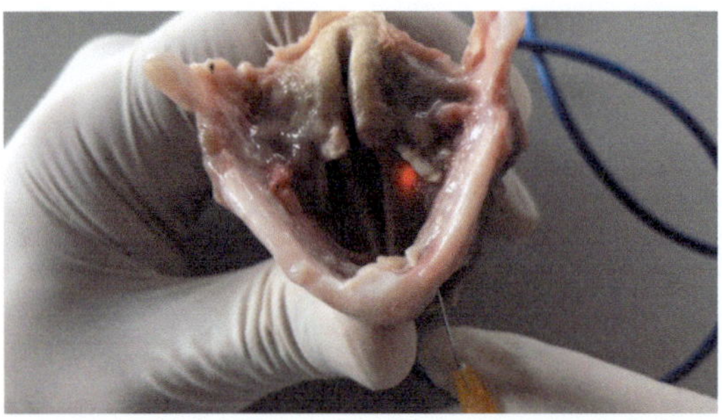

Fig. 6.8 Laser guided identification of the needle tip in a canine larynx. The location of the needle tip is precisely indicated and the depth of the needle can be approximated by observing the brightness and size of the laser spot. (Figure courtesy of Dr. Wonjae Cha)

6.3 Conclusion

Trans-CT approach for vocal fold injection under local anesthesia at the outpatient clinic is a safe and effective technique for variety of purposes. Short extramucosal route of this approach provides better patient's compliance but its blind nature necessitates a steep learning curve for successful results. Surgeons should be versed with detailed techniques to overcome the limitations.

Key Learning Points:

- Trans-CT approach is a fast and simple way for vocal fold injection after the initial learning curve.
- Endoscopic visualization of anterior subglottis enables surgeons to identify CT membrane even in patients with poor surgical landmarks.
- Precise identification of inferior border of the thyroid cartilage is critical in estimating the level of true vocal fold. "Walking down technique" is the most effective strategy for this purpose.
- Careful palpation with the needle within the vocal fold provides sufficient information of the needle depth and location.

References

1. Seifert A. Percutaneous paraffin injection to eliminate the effects of unilateral laryngeal paralysis. Z Laryngol Rhinol Otol Ihre Grenzgeb. 1916:233–5.
2. Ward PH, Hanson DG, Abemayor E. Transcutaneous Teflon injection of the paralyzed vocal cord: a new technique. Laryngoscope. 1985;95(6):644–9. https://doi.org/10.1288/00005537-198506000-00002.

3. Hirano M, Tanaka S, Tanaka Y, Hibi S. Transcutaneous intrafold injection for unilateral vocal fold paralysis: functional results. Ann Otol Rhinol Laryngol. 1990;99(8):598–604. https://doi.org/10.1177/000348949009900802.
4. Mallur PS, Rosen CA. Vocal fold injection: review of indications, techniques, and materials for augmentation. Clin Exp Otorhinolaryngol. 2010;3(4):177.
5. Cha W, Ro JH, Wang SG, Jang JY, Cho JK, Kim GH, et al. Development of a device for real-time light-guided vocal fold injection: a preliminary report. Laryngoscope. 2016;126(4):936–40.
6. Chhetri DK, Jamal N. Percutaneous injection laryngoplasty. Laryngoscope. 2014;124(3):742–5. https://doi.org/10.1002/lary.24417.
7. Clary MS, Milam BM, Courey MS. Office-based vocal fold injection with the laryngeal introducer technique. Laryngoscope. 2014;124(9):2114–7. https://doi.org/10.1002/lary.24659.
8. Hoffman HT, Dailey SH, Bock JM, Thibeault SL, McCulloch TM. Transillumination for needle localization in the larynx. Laryngoscope. 2015;125(10):2341–8. https://doi.org/10.1002/lary.25372.
9. Jin SM, Park CY, Lee JK, Ban JH, Lee SH, Lee KC. Transcutaneous injection laryngoplasty through the cricothyroid space in the sitting position: anatomical information and technique. European archives of oto-rhino-laryngology. 2008;265(3):313–9. doi: https://doi.org/10.1007/s00405-007-0450-6.
10. Gotxi-Erezuma I, Ortega-Galán M, Laso-Elguezabal A, Prieto Puga G, Bullido-Alonso C, García-Gutiérrez S, et al. Electromyography-guided hyaluronic acid injection laryngoplasty in early stage of unilateral vocal fold paralysis. Acta Otorrinolaringol Esp. 2017;68(5):274–83. https://doi.org/10.1016/j.otorri.2016.12.001.
11. Wang CC, Chang MH, Jiang RS, Lai HC, De Virgilio A, Wang CP, et al. Laryngeal electromyography-guided hyaluronic acid vocal fold injection for unilateral vocal fold paralysis: a prospective long-term follow-up outcome report. JAMA Otolaryngol Head Neck Surg. 2015;141(3):264–71. https://doi.org/10.1001/jamaoto.2014.3466.

7 Trans-Thyrohyoid Approach

Jin Ho Sohn

Abstract

Trans-thyrohyoid approach is a percutaneous vocal fold injection technique in which a needle is inserted through the thyrohyoid membrane between the thyroid cartilage and the hyoid bone to reach the vocal fold. Throughout the procedure, the needle is visible; hence the procedure is relatively simple and straightforward to perform. This approach also allows for easy access to the vocal folds, so even patients under local anesthesia demonstrate great tolerance.

Keywords

Trans-thyrohyoid approach · Thyrohyoid membrane · Percutaneous vocal fold injection Injection laryngoplasty

Trans-thyrohyoid (TH) approach is a percutaneous vocal fold injection technique in which a needle is inserted through the thyrohyoid membrane and injected into the vocal fold.

TH approach is one of the most recently introduced techniques among the vocal fold injection methods currently in use. In 2005, Getz et al. first introduced the TH approach when injecting Cidofovir for a recurrent papilloma arising in the supraglottis [1]. In 2006, Amin reported that TH approach led to successful vocal fold injections for vocal fold augmentations for the 10 patients evaluated in his retrospective chart review [2].

7.1 Technique

7.1.1 Procedure

The local anesthesia method is identical to other approaches, except that anesthesia is additionally required for both the skin and subcutaneous tissues overlying the thyrohyoid membrane. Procedurally, after administering the local anesthetics, the assistant inserts a flexible videoendoscope transnasally and positions it to allow for adequate visualization of the larynx including the lower portion of the epiglottis to confirm needle positioning. While the patient maintains a slight neck-extended posture, the surgeon locates both the hyoid bone and the superior notch of thyroid cartilage by palpation and then inserts the needle between them. As the needle is pushed through the thyrohyoid membrane, make sure to direct the tip downwards to gently advance through the preepiglottic space. Watching the monitor, the surgeon makes sure that the needle enters the laryngeal cavity through the petiole of the epiglottis and then places and inserts the needle tip into the desired vocal fold area to administer the injection (Fig. 7.1).

J. H. Sohn (✉)
Department of Otolaryngology-Head and Neck Surgery, Kyungpook National University Chilgok Hospital, Daegu, South Korea

© Springer Nature Singapore Pte Ltd. 2021

B.-J. Lee et al. (eds.), *Vocal Fold Injection*, https://doi.org/10.1007/978-981-16-3303-4_7

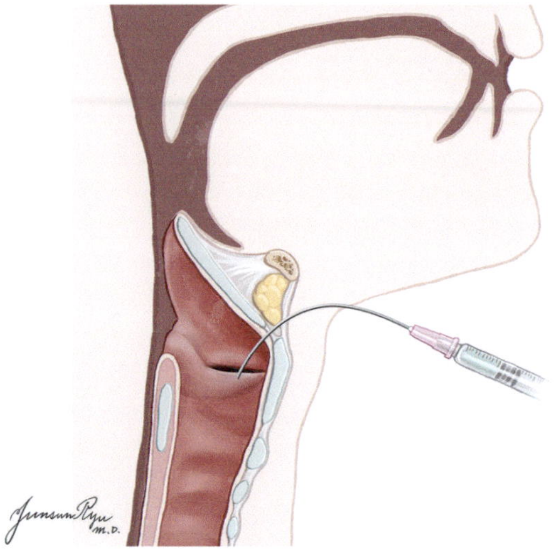

Fig. 7.1 Trans-thyrohyoid vocal fold injection

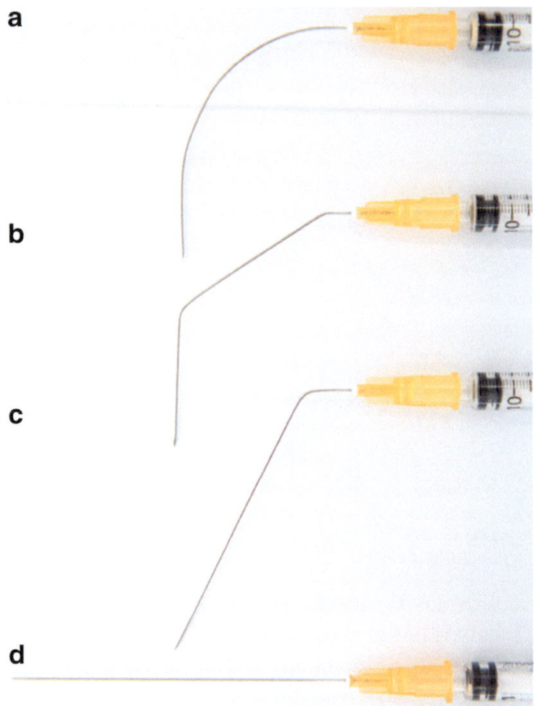

Fig. 7.2 Various needle shapes used for trans-thyrohyoid approach. (**a**) Gently curved needle, bent 90°. (**b**) Double-bend needle. (**c**) Bend needle from 45° to 90° near the hub. (**d**) Straight needle

7.1.2 Needle Preparations

The distance between the neck skin to the vocal cords is longer than that of the trans-cricothryoid, thus basing on the author's experience, the needle should be at least 2 in.-long. As for the needle thickness, it may vary depending on the material being injected, but for injecting general fillers, botulinum toxin, or steroid, a 24–25 gauge is commonly used.

Although documents recommend using a 1.5-in. needle [2, 3], it is not long enough to reach the injection site in large larynges [4]. In addition, when considering the anatomical structure, bending the needle will allow for a smoother access to the vocal folds. Achkar et al. recommend using a double-bend needle [3], and Dion and Neklsen recommend using a bent needle of 45–90° near the hub [5]. Some practitioners, including the author, recommend using a gently curved needle, bent 90° [6] (Fig. 7.2). Some others recommend using a straight needle [2, 7]; however, based on the author's experience, using it could be difficult to reach the anterior vocal fold because the mandible may interfere with the injection process.

7.1.3 Technical Tips

While reports state that accessing the anterior vocal fold is difficult using the trans-thyrohyoid approach [4, 8, 9], when the needle is properly bent and used skillfully by an experienced practitioner, the anterior vocal fold is accessed without a problem in most cases. In order to make it easier to aim the needle toward the desired vocal fold area, the needle should enter the laryngeal cavity through the petiole of the epiglottis close to the vocal folds. In other words, if the needle enters the laryngeal cavity through the epiglottis cartilage far from the vocal fold, it will be difficult to adjust its direction due to the rigidity of the cartilage. On the other hand, when the needle enters the laryngeal cavity through the soft and elastic region—where there is no cartilage

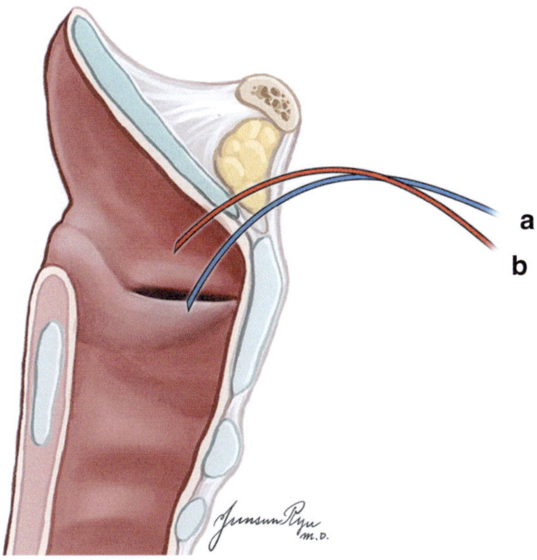

Fig. 7.3 Technical tips. (**a**) When the needle enters the laryngeal cavity through the soft and elastic region—where there is no cartilage between the lower border of the epiglottic cartilage and vocal folds—it will be easier to control its direction afterwards. (**b**) Otherwise, if the needle pierces the epiglottis cartilage, it will be difficult to adjust its direction due to the rigidity of the cartilage

between the lower border of the epiglottic cartilage and vocal folds—it will be easier to control its direction afterwards (Fig. 7.3).

Nevertheless, in the case that the needle cannot access the desired vocal fold area, the laryngeal introducer technique proposed by Clary et al. may be helpful [4]. The laryngeal introducer technique involves first, inserting a thick and strong 1.5-in. 18G needle into the laryngeal cavity; next, inserting a 3.5-in. 25G spinal needle into the lumen of the needle; and then using the strong rigidity of the thick introducer needle for the injection needle to reach the desired vocal fold area.

While this technique is helpful for reaching the target injection area, the author indicates that the procedure of inserting a thin injecting needle through the introducer needle is quite cumbersome and time-consuming. This can, in fact, possibly result in bleeding from the puncture site, which will make both the patient and the surgeon uncomfortable. Based on the author's experience, it is much easier and quicker to execute the injection procedure when a thin injection needle is inserted into the introducer needle prior to the procedure. The injection needle tip must not exceed the introducer needle tip before inserting the introducer needle to the laryngeal cavity. Only after the introducer needle enters the laryngeal cavity, should the injection needle pass through the introducer needle to reach the laryngeal cavity and be injected into the target site. The author also reports that it is easier to handle the 25G needle with 2.5 in. rather than 3.5 in. Additionally, the 18 gauge introducer needle has strong enough rigidity to adjust its direction freely in the larynx bent only 45° compared to the 25 gauge used for conventional TH approach that is bent 90° (Fig. 7.4).

As described above, most injections are conducted only with a thin needle. However, the laryngeal introducer technique can be an alternative method for surgeons inexperienced as well as for some cases that are difficult to treat using only a thin needle.

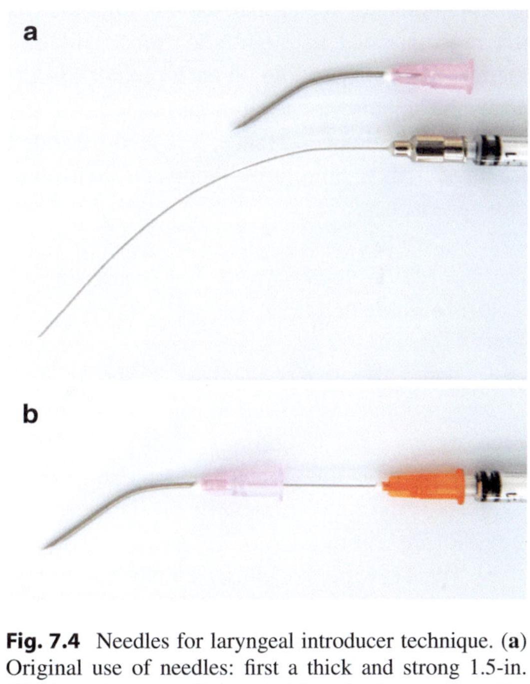

Fig. 7.4 Needles for laryngeal introducer technique. (**a**) Original use of needles: first a thick and strong 1.5-in. 18G introducer needle inserted into the laryngeal cavity, then a 3.5 in. 25G spinal injection needle inserted through the lumen of the needle. (**b**) Modified use of needles: a thin 2.5-in. injection needle inserted into the introducer needle prior to the procedure

7.2 Advantages and Limitations

Unlike trans-cricothyroid approach and trans-cartilaginous approach, TH approach allows consistent needle visibility throughout the procedure. Therefore, the needle can be easily adjusted and brought to the target area [2, 4, 6, 7]. Furthermore with the TH approach, both sides of the vocal fold can be injected with a single needle insertion [2], and the supraglottic area can easily be accessed for injection. Even though some minor bleeding at the puncture site of the epiglottis may occur, it would not be considered an obstacle to the overall procedure. In some, no serious complications have been reported with TH approach [6].

There are no specific contraindications or limitations in performing TH approach. Nonetheless, in cases where the patient's hyoid bone and thyroid cartilage is impalpable due to small laryngeal framework or obesity, it may be difficult to implement the technique, especially for women patients.

This does not mean that the TH approach is the most optimal method. The 'most suitable' method varies depending on each patient's tolerance and anatomical limitations as well as the surgeon's preferences. Hence, it is recommended for physicians to familiarize themselves with several approaches.

Key Learning Points:

- Trans-thyrohyoid (TH) approach is a percutaneous injection technique in which a needle is inserted through the thyrohyoid membrane to reach the vocal fold or several various sites in the larynx for injection.
- The TH approach allows for a facilitated access to the target vocal fold area as the needle is visible throughout the procedure. Once inserted, the needle can inject injectables into both vocal folds.
- The recommendation is to use needles 2 in. or longer and that the needle should be bent for use.
- When the needle enters the laryngeal cavity, inserting it through the petiole of the epiglottis close to the vocal fold without piercing the epiglottic cartilage will make it easier to target the desired vocal fold.
- If the needle entering the laryngeal cavity cannot target the desired vocal cord area well, then trying the laryngeal introducer technique may help.

References

1. Getz AE, Scharf J, Amin MR. Thyrohyoid approach to cidofovir injection: a case study. J Voice. 2005;19:501–3.
2. Amin MR. Thyrohyoid approach for vocal fold augmentation. Ann Otol Rhinol Laryngol. 2006;115:699–702.
3. Achkar J, Song P, Andrus J, Franco R Jr. Double-bend needle modification for Transthyrohyoid vocal fold injection. Laryngoscope. 2012;122:865–7.
4. Clary MS, Milam BM, Courey MS. Office-based vocal fold injection with the laryngeal introducer technique. Laryngoscope. 2014;124:2114–7.
5. Dion GR, Nielsen SW. In-office laryngology injections. Otolaryngol Clin N Am. 2019;52(3):521–36.
6. Woo SH, Son YI, Lee SH, Park JJ, Kim YP. Comparative analysis on the efficiency of the injection Laryngoplasty technique using calcium hydroxyapatite (CaHA): the thyrohyoid approach versus the cricothyroid approach. J Voice. 2013;27(2):236–41.
7. Mallur PS, Rosen CA. Office-based laryngeal injections. Otolaryngol Clin N Am. 2013;46:85–100.
8. Zeitler D, Amin MR. The thyrohyoid approach to in-office injection augmentation of the vocal fold. Curr Opin Otolaryngol Head Neck Surg. 2007;15:412–6.
9. Sulica L, Rosen CA, Postma GN, et al. Current practice in injection augmentation of the vocal folds: indications, treatment principles, techniques, and complications. Laryngoscope. 2010;120:319–25.

8 Trans-Cartilaginous Approach

Seung-Won Lee

Abstract

Injection laryngoplasty (IL) has gained popularity in recent years as a method to manage unilateral vocal cord paralysis and vocal fold atrophy [1]. Various transcutaneous approaches can be used to access the vocal folds, such as through the cricothyroid (CT) membrane and thyrohyoid (TH) membrane, as well as directly through thyroid cartilage.

Each approach has advantages and disadvantages. Familiarity with these approaches allows the surgeon to tailor the procedure to patient anatomy and may provide better voice results. The transcartilaginous (TC) approach allows augmentation of the anterior vocal fold and direct puncture of the thyroid cartilage at the level of the vocal folds. The TC approach may be a useful alternative when the CT and TH approaches are not possible and may obtain optimal voice results. In addition, when augmentation of the anterior vocal fold is insufficient after CT or TH approach injection, the TC approach could be performed in combination with either approach to obtain optimal results.

Keywords

Injection laryngoplasty · Thyroid cartilage
Transcartilaginous approach · Vocal folds

8.1 Injection Laryngoplasty Techniques in Korea

According to a 2009 survey of Korean phonosurgeons about injection laryngoplasty (IL) techniques, the cricothyroid (CT) approach is the most commonly performed percutaneous IL approach, followed by the transcartilaginous (TC) approach. When the CT approach is not possible, the TC and thyrohyoid (TH) approaches may be useful alternatives (Fig. 8.1) [2].

8.2 Transcartilaginous Approach Procedure

All IL procedures with the TC approach are performed percutaneously under local anesthesia. Before the procedure, the patient inhales 4% lidocaine through a nebulizer for 10 min. A spray catheter with a flexible fiberscope is used to apply a 4% lidocaine solution onto the vocal folds [2, 3].

Surgeons may use different needle gauges depending on the type of injection material. Typically, a 25-gauge disposable needle is used to administer hyaluronic acid derivatives, or a

S.-W. Lee (✉)
Department of Otolaryngology Head and Neck Surgery, Soonchunhyang University College of Medicine, Bucheon, South Korea
e-mail: lsw0922@schmc.ac.kr

© Springer Nature Singapore Pte Ltd. 2021

B.-J. Lee et al. (eds.), *Vocal Fold Injection*, https://doi.org/10.1007/978-981-16-3303-4_8

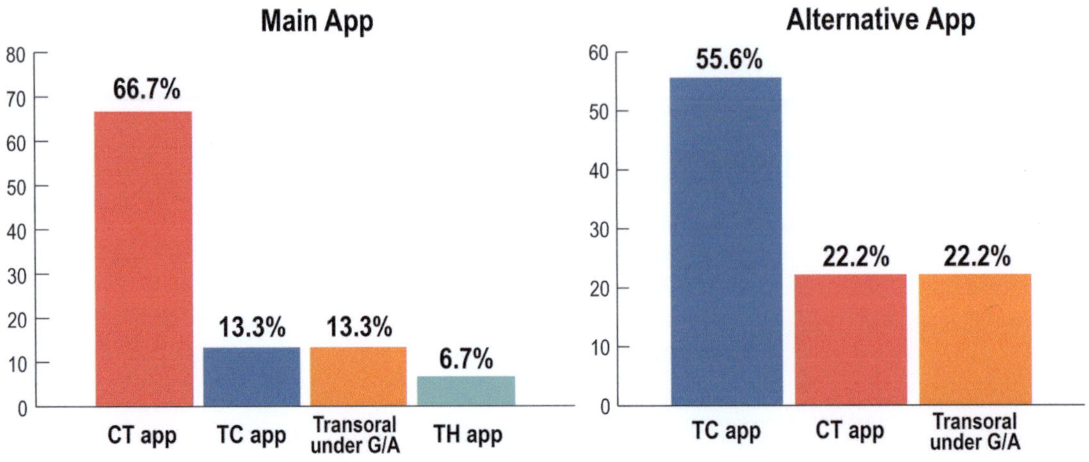

Fig. 8.1 Main and alternative approaches for injection laryngoplasty; results of a survey of Korean phonosurgeons

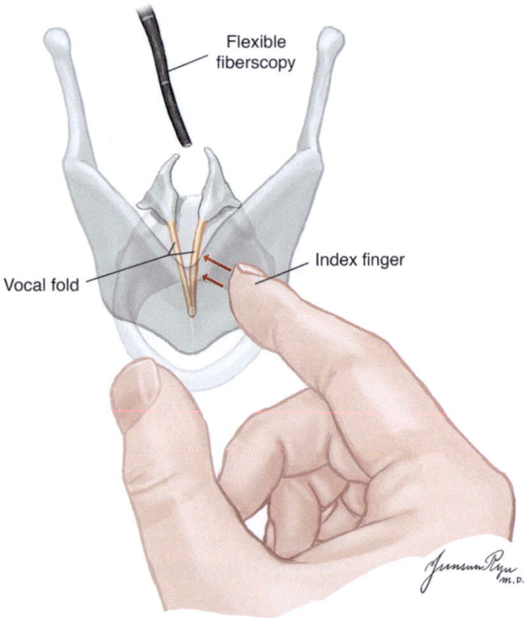

Fig. 8.2 Confirmation of the vocal fold level to press the thyroid cartilage

22-gauge disposable needle is used to administer calcium hydroxyapatite materials.

The vocal folds are located at one-half of the height of the thyroid cartilage in men, and at one-third in women. However, it is important to check the actual vocal fold level by pressing the thyroid cartilage and confirming passive vocal fold movement (Fig. 8.2) [4].

A digital trans-nasal flexible fiberscope is used to confirm appropriate needle location, which is 0.5–1.0 cm lateral to the vocal folds. For the TC approach, the thyroid cartilage is directly punctured, just inferior to its halfway point. The tip of the needle is visible submucosally and is withdrawn slightly to administer the injection. The injection is administered slowly to the vocalis muscle in front of the vocal process; injection is continued until slight overcorrection is achieved. For anterior vocal fold augmentation with the TC approach, the injection is administered toward the midline at the vocal fold level; for posterior vocal fold augmentation, the injection is administered away from the midline (Fig. 8.3). After injection, check the patient's glottal contact and voice improvement, and then complete the procedure.

8.3 Other Uses of the Transcartilaginous Approach

If laryngeal electromyography is unavailable, the surgeon can use the point-touch technique to check laryngeal anatomy with the fingers before performing the TC approach [5]. A flexible fiberscope or the point-touch technique is used to confirm patient anatomy before injection of botulinum toxin into the thyroarytenoid muscle.

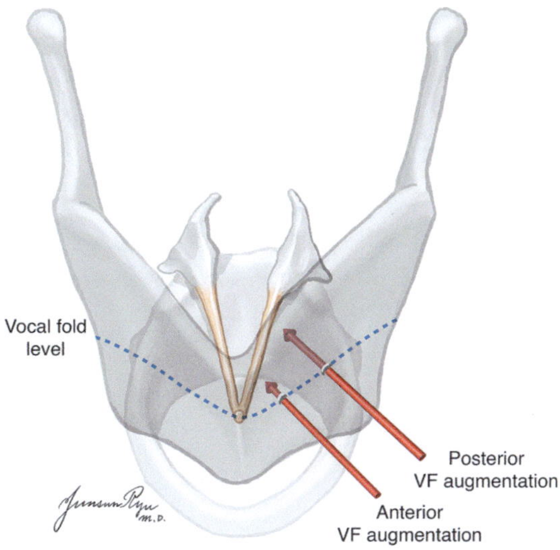

Fig. 8.3 Direction of injection with the transcartilaginous approach for vocal fold augmentation. For anterior vocal fold augmentation, material is injected toward the midline at the vocal fold level; for posterior vocal fold augmentation, material is injected away from the midline

Because diffuse administration of botulinum toxin is effective, precise injection into the exact thyroarytenoid muscle is not necessary. Percutaneous steroid injection for benign vocal fold lesions can also be performed with the TC approach [6]. The TC approach may be appropriate because such lesions are anterior to the middle membranous vocal fold and within the subepithelial or Reinke's space. Decide to use the TC or CT approach for percutaneous steroid injection on the basis of patient's anatomy and lesions (Fig. 8.4) [7].

8.4 Advantages and Disadvantages the Transcartilaginous Approach

The TC approach has many advantages. (1) The working distance is short because the thyroid cartilage is directly punctured [5]. (2) Injection is administered at the vocal fold level; moreover, the approach is parallel, not oblique, to the vocal fold level. (3) The targeted area is easily located and the depth of injection is easy to control. (4) The TC approach is useful for patients with problematic anatomical landmarks, such as those with previous neck treatments and those with a narrow CT space due to congenital and postoperative causes [8] (5) Finally, the TC approach is a good alternative when the CT approach is impossible (Fig. 8.5).

The TC approach also has two disadvantages. (1) For some patients, the TC approach is contraindicated because ossification of the thyroid cartilage prevents passage of the needle through the thyroid cartilage; thus, the CT or TH approach may be required. (2) The cartilage matrix may plug the needle lumen if the surgeon cannot determine the appropriate location in the vocal folds for the needle. If this happens, considerable force is required for injection, or the needle must be changed [4].

8.5 Technical Pitfalls of the Transcartilaginous Approach

In general, a smaller volume of material is injected with the TC approach compared to that of the CT approach. For the TC approach, the needle is directly inserted into the thyroid cartilage parallel to the vocal folds; for the CT approach, the needle is inserted from the bottom and through the paraglottic space. In my study, the mean volume of injection with the TC approach (0.65 ± 0.2 mL) was significantly less than that of the CT approach (0.84 ± 0.27 mL). Therefore, the effects achieved with the TC approach may subside faster than those of the CT approach.

After direct puncture of thyroid cartilage, the surgeon must control the depth of injection. Superficial injection into Reinke's space may worsen voice outcomes. The cartilage matrix may plug the needle lumen, as several attempts may be needed to penetrate the thyroid cartilage and initiate injection, and considerable force may be needed to inject the material; therefore, excessive material may be injected into the vocal folds. To avoid this problem, disposable needles should be changed when needed.

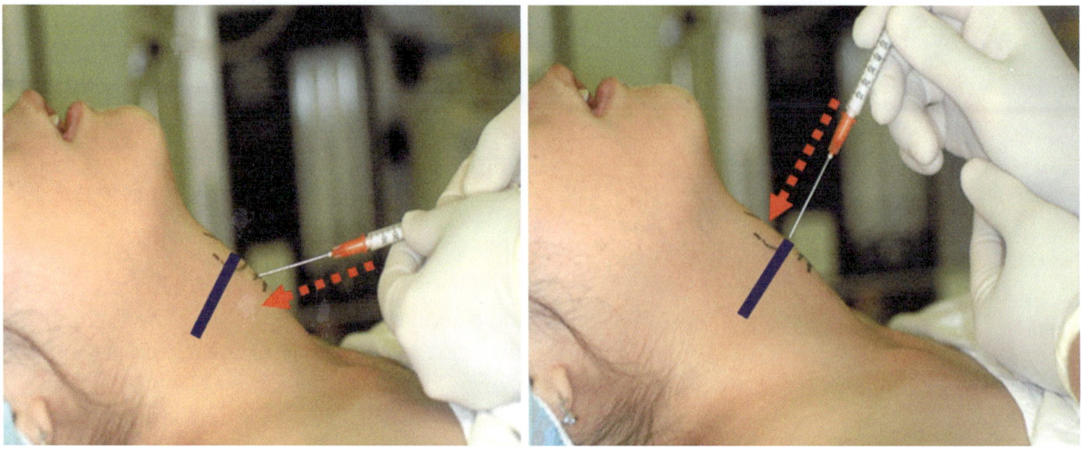

Fig. 8.4 Transcartilaginous vs cricothyroid approach

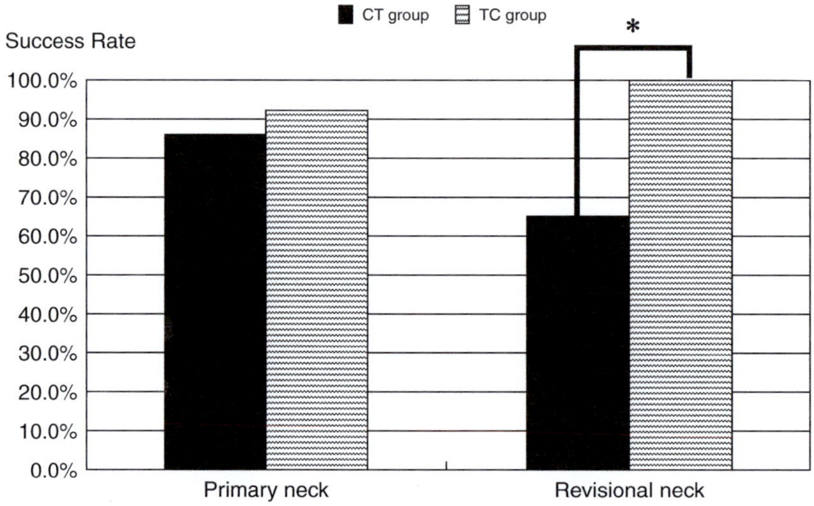

Fig. 8.5 Success rates of the transcartilaginous (TC) and cricothyroid (CT) approaches. The success rate of the TC approach was significantly greater than that of the CT approach (100% vs 65%, respectively) for revisional neck group [8]. *Primary neck* consisted of patients who did not undergo neck surgery before injection. *Revisional neck* consisted of patients who underwent neck surgery before injection. *Significant difference between the CT and TC approach groups

Key Learning Points:

- The TC approach is a one of the transcutaneous IL techniques.
- The TC approach is used to penetrate the thyroid cartilage directly; therefore, the working distance is short, and the anterior vocal fold is easily located.
- The TC approach is useful for patients with problematic anatomical landmarks, such as those with previous neck treatment and a narrow CT space.
- If a single IL procedure performed with the CT or TH approach does not achieve complete glottal contact with the anterior vocal fold, the TC approach could be used to achieve better voice results.

References

1. Kwon TK, Buckmire R. Injection laryngoplasty for management of unilateral vocal fold paralysis. Curr Opin Otolaryngol Head Neck Surg. 2004;12:538–42.
2. Lee SWK, J. W., Koh YW, Lee JH. Premedication & anesthesia for OPD based laryngeal procedures. J Korean Soc Laryngol Phoniatr Logoped. 2009;20:11–6.
3. Lee SW, Son YI, Kim CH, Lee JY, Kim SC, Koh YW. Voice outcomes of polyacrylamide hydrogel injection laryngoplasty. Laryngoscope. 2007;117:1871–5.
4. Jin SM, Park CY, Lee JK, Ban JH, Lee SH, Lee KC. Transcutaneous injection laryngoplasty through the cricothyroid space in the sitting position: anatomical information and technique. Eur Arch Otorhinolaryngol. 2008;265:313–9.
5. Green DC, Berke GS, Ward PH, Gerratt BR. Point-touch technique of botulinum toxin injection for the treatment of spasmodic dysphonia. Ann Otol Rhinol Laryngol. 1992;101:883–7.
6. Lee SW, Park KN. Long-term efficacy of percutaneous steroid injection for treating benign vocal fold lesions: a prospective study. Laryngoscope. 2016;126:2315–9.
7. Woo JH, Kim DY, Kim JW, Oh EA, Lee SW. Efficacy of percutaneous vocal fold injections for benign laryngeal lesions: prospective multicenter study. Acta Otolaryngol. 2011;131:1326–32.
8. Lee SW, Kim JW, Koh YW, Shim SS, Son YI. Comparative analysis of efficiency of injection Laryngoplasty technique for with or without neck treatment patients: a Transcartilaginous approach versus the cricothyroid approach. Clin Exp Otorhinolaryngol. 2010;3:37–41.

Part III

Considerations in Immobile Vocal Folds

Optimal Injection Timing for Vocal Fold Paralysis

9

Seung-Ho Choi

Abstract

Vocal fold (VF) immobility, in a narrow sense, VF paralysis causes symptoms of breathy voice, loss of vocal pitch and loudness, shortness of breath and aspiration. VF paralysis may be temporary, and recovery of the function varies depending on the type and location of the nerve injury. Regardless of the cause or prognosis, injection laryngoplasty is effective in improving symptoms of VF paralysis. Injection material is selected in consideration of the duration of paralysis and the possibility of recovery. If the patient has high vocal demand or aspiration, early injection laryngoplasty is favorable. Early injection tends to lower the need for later framework surgery and improve the final voice quality. Injection laryngoplasty with permanent material is generally recommended when the nerve injury has been confirmed by electromyography or during the surgery, or after waiting for recovery for at least 6 months, although some reports indicated that the permanent injection material did not adversely affect the natural recovery.

S.-H. Choi (✉)
Department of Otorhinolaryngology-Head and Neck Surgery, Asan Medical Center, University of Ulsan College of Medicine, Seoul, South Korea
e-mail: shchoi@amc.seoul.kr

Keywords

Vocal fold immobility · Vocal fold paralysis Recurrent laryngeal nerve · Injection laryngoplasty · Phonosurgery

VF immobility refers to a condition in which the movement of the vocal folds is reduced, and the term VF paralysis is often used interchangeably although diagnosis of VF paralysis should be made only when paralysis is confirmed through electromyography or when damage of the recurrent laryngeal nerve is confirmed. Besides recurrent laryngeal nerve paralysis, VF immobility may result from various situations including cricoarytenoid joint subluxation/dislocation caused by trauma, cricoarytenoid joint arthritis and fixation caused by systemic disorders, neoplastic condition that hinders the VF mobility, etc. Signs and symptoms of VF immobility include breathy voice, loss of vocal pitch and loudness, shortness of breath while speaking, and choking or coughing while swallowing food, drink or saliva. Paralysis of recurrent laryngeal nerve can show varying degrees of symptoms and the possibility of recovery depending on the degree of nerve damage.

Whatever the situation, if the vocal folds do not close sufficiently, injection laryngoplasty may help. Technological changes including high definition flexible endoscopy, injection material that can be passed through a small needle, and trans-oral and transcutaneous injection technique

© Springer Nature Singapore Pte Ltd. 2021

B.-J. Lee et al. (eds.), *Vocal Fold Injection*, https://doi.org/10.1007/978-981-16-3303-4_9

have rapidly changed the management of unilateral VF paralysis. In the past, laryngeal framework surgery such as type I thyroplasty or arytenoid adduction was the mainstay of VF paralysis treatment, but injection laryngoplasty has become most popular for last 2 decades.

9.1 Natural History of VF Paralysis

Neural regeneration depends on the type, extent and location of the nerve damage. Once a peripheral nerve is damaged, the distal portion of the axon that is disconnected from the cell body undergoes fragmentation and decomposition which is called Wallerian degeneration. If the endoneurium is intact, the proximal axon can regenerate and reinnervate the target muscle, allowing recovery of function. With neurapraxia or axonotmesis, complete recovery can be expected over a varying period of time, but if the nerve is completely divided (neurotmesis) or severely disorganized, symptoms are severe and permanent. The location of nerve damage is also important for symptoms and prognosis. If the recurrent laryngeal nerve is injured just before the entrance to the larynx, e.g., during thyroid surgery, symptoms may be limited to hoarseness and aspiration, but if high vagal paralysis occurs after skull base surgery, pharyngeal hyposensation and severe dysphagia can occur due to superior laryngeal nerve paralysis as well. Because the axonal regeneration is a slow process and skeletal muscles become atrophic and fibrous after a long-time denervation, reinnervation does not necessarily imply restoration of function, and time is a very important factor in determining the prognosis of VF paralysis. Consequently, identification of the cause of VF paralysis in a specific patient and knowledge of natural history of VF paralysis is of paramount importance to predict prognosis and determine treatment. According to Sulica's meta-analysis report, complete recovery of motion occurred in 36 ± 22% (range 13–83%) of idiopathic VF paralysis, and if partial recovery was included, the rate increased to 39 ± 20% (range, 19–83%) [1]. Complete recovery of voice occurred in 52 ± 17% (range, 25–87%) of cases, some degree of recovery in 61 ± 22% (range, 25–87%). Most of the recovery tended to occur within 1 year, and only a small subset of patients recovered later. However, the author concluded there was marked variation in rates of recovery among reports because of variations in definitions of recovery, oversimplified all-or-none notions of paralysis and recovery, and inconsistent reporting of time elapsed from onset of paralysis to evaluation. Husain et al. reported a 69% recovery rate of vocal function among 55 idiopathic unilateral VF paralysis [2]. The mean time to recovery was 152.8 ± 109.3 days, and two-thirds of patients recovered within 6 months. Age, gender, laterality, use of injection augmentation did not influence recovery rate. The authors recommended to consider framework surgery after 6 months because of the declining probability of recovery over time. Rubin et al. conducted a study comparing idiopathic VF paralysis and non-idiopathic non-traumatic VF paralysis [3]. Although diagnostic errors including problems such as upper respiratory tract infection, immunosuppression, and malignant tumors were found in the idiopathic VF paralysis group, the 5-year actuarial estimate for recovery differed significantly: 53.2% in idiopathic group versus 17.9% in non-idiopathic non-traumatic group. Mau et al. performed a research predicting recovery after VF paralysis by mathematical modeling [4]. Of 727 cases of unilateral VF paralysis over a 7 year period, 44 reported spontaneous recovery with a discrete onset of vocal improvement. The authors showed a bimodal peak in the probability distribution of the recovery of VF motion, one peak at 3–4 months and the other at 12 months. Cumulative probabilities of vocal recovery were 65.9%, 85.6%, 96.0%, 98.9% and 99.9% at 4 months, 6 months, 9 months, 12 months, 18 months, respectively. Earlier vocal recovery was associated with recovery of VF motion and younger age. The authors concluded that waiting 12 months for spontaneous recovery was probably too conservative.

9.2 Optimal Injection Timing

In the past when injection laryngoplasty was not popular, the treatment of VF paralysis was limited to surgery such as type I thyroplasty or arytenoid addition. An observation period of 6 months to 1 year before surgery was generally recommended and wait-and-see policy for spontaneous recovery or compensation was considered a reasonable option. However, as high-resolution videoendoscopy and various injection materials with various duration of efficacy have been developed, injection laryngoplasty can be easily performed in an outpatient clinic under local anesthesia. Therefore, the management strategy of VF paralysis became quite different from the past [5]. In addition, injection laryngoplasty is rarely excluded even in patients who are deemed unsuitable for general anesthesia or invasive surgery, and now play an essential role in palliative management of these terminal patients with VF paralysis.

VF paralysis usually go through a process of compensation to various degrees. Some patients get well quickly after rapid compensation, while others experience long-lasting severe symptoms despite compensation. Excessive activity of the suprahyoid muscles and the contralateral VF causes laryngeal elevation, contraction of the supraglottis, and hyperadduction of the contralateral VF and resultant glottal closure [6]. The need for injection laryngoplasty has to be determined by the patient's situation: current symptom requiring immediate treatment, progress of compensation, and prospects on recovery. If symptoms are mild and early recovery is expected, injection laryngoplasty may not be necessary. In the case of patients with high voice demand or with dysphonia or aspiration that interfere with daily life, it is desirable to perform injection laryngoplasty as soon as possible regardless of the possibility of recovery. In particular, if the cause of the paralysis is direct nerve damage during thoracic surgery or skull base surgery, early injection laryngoplasty is recommended because the patient's pulmonary and airway protection function is severely declined or high vagal paralysis has the potential to cause life-threatening aspiration pneumonia [7, 8].

Several authors reported that early injection laryngoplasty reduced the need for later framework surgery and had the advantage of better voice quality. Friedman et al. reported that 62% of patients who underwent injection within 6 months maintained adequate voice compared with none who received late injection [9]. They concluded that early injection laryngoplasty with hyaluronic acid decreased the need for transcervical medialization laryngoplasty in patients with VF paralysis. Fang et al. reported a prospective cohort study to determine which patients with VF paralysis ultimately needed permanent laryngoplasty [10]. They concluded that wider initial glottal gap was a robust early predictor of permanent laryngoplasty, and early injection laryngoplasty could reduce the need for permanent laryngoplasty in patients with a large glottal gap.

Key Learning Points:

- Injection laryngoplasty is effective in improving symptoms of VF paralysis regardless of the cause or prognosis.
- Early injection laryngoplasty is preferable especially for patients with high vocal demand or aspiration.
- Injection laryngoplasty with permanent material is generally recommended when the nerve injury has been confirmed or after waiting for recovery for at least 6 months.

References

1. Sulica L. The natural history of idiopathic unilateral vocal fold paralysis: evidence and problems. Laryngoscope. 2008;118(7):1303–7.
2. Husain S, Sadoughi B, Mor N, Levin AM, Sulica L. Time course of recovery of idiopathic vocal fold paralysis. Laryngoscope. 2018;128(1):148–52.
3. Rubin F, Villeneuve A, Alciato L, Slaim L, Bonfils P, Laccourreye O. Idiopathic unilateral vocal-fold paralysis in the adult. Eur Ann Otorhinolaryngol Head Neck Dis. 2018;135(3):171–4.
4. Mau T, Pan HM, Childs LF. The natural history of recoverable vocal fold paralysis: implications for kinetics of reinnervation. Laryngoscope. 2017;127(11):2585–90.
5. Costello D. Change to earlier surgical interventions: contemporary management of unilateral vocal fold paralysis. Curr Opin Otolaryngol Head Neck Surg. 2015;23(3):181–4.
6. Xu X, Zhuang P, Wilson A, Jiang JJ. Compensatory movement of contralateral vocal folds in patients with unilateral vocal fold paralysis. J Voice. 2019;1997(19):30323–6.
7. Anderson TD, Mirza N. Immediate percutaneous medialization for acute vocal fold immobility with aspiration. Laryngoscope. 2001;111(8):1318–21.
8. Graboyes EM, Bradley JP, Meyers BF, Nussenbaum B. Efficacy and safety of acute injection laryngoplasty for vocal cord paralysis following thoracic surgery. Laryngoscope. 2011;121(11):2406–10.
9. Friedman AD, Burns JA, Heaton JT, Zeitels SM. Early versus late injection medialization for unilateral vocal cord paralysis. Laryngoscope. 2010;120(10):2042–6.
10. Fang TJ, Pei YC, Li HY, Wong AM, Chiang HC. Glottal gap as an early predictor for permanent laryngoplasty in unilateral vocal fold paralysis. Laryngoscope. 2014;124(9):2125–30.

Ideal Material Selection for Vocal Fold Augmentation

10

Thomas L. Carroll

Abstract

The ideal material for a vocal fold injection augmentation for unilateral vocal fold immobility depends on the immobile vocal fold's likelihood to recover function through natural nerve healing. In cases of permanent immobility from an issue related to arytenoid joint pathology or paralysis due to a neurologic injury or illness, durable or permanent materials are chosen. Shorter acting augmentation materials can be utilized in the setting of immobility when (1) the permanence of the condition is yet to be determined, or (2) due to coexisting other glottic pathology, the outcome of unilateral injection augmentation is unclear (Mallur and Rosen. Clin Exp Otorhinolaryngol. 3(4):177-82; 2010). This chapter will cover the materials available for vocal fold augmentation, focusing on non-autologous injectables that are available "off-the-shelf."

T. L. Carroll (✉)
Department of Otolaryngology-Head and Neck Surgery, Harvard Medical School, Boston, MA, USA

Division of Otolaryngology, Department of Surgery, Brigham and Women's Hospital, Boston, MA, USA
e-mail: tcarroll@bwh.harvard.edu

Keywords

Calcium Hydroxylapatite
Carboxymethylcellulose · Hyaluronic acid
Silk · Polydimethylsiloxane

10.1 Material Selection

Choosing an appropriate material for injection augmentation requires a knowledge of (1) the available materials' durations of effect, (2) the prognosis of the vocal fold (VF) for eventual recovery of motion, and/or (3) the patient's prognosis for survival (and thus their ability to return for subsequent augmentation). The injectables discussed below will be those available off-the-shelf for injection augmentation (IA) and not autologous materials such as fat or fascia (see Chap. 11).

While not a hard and fast rule, in the setting of a VF immobility less than 6 months from the time of onset or one being followed by laryngeal EMG with potential for recovery (no synkinesis, evidence of improved prognosis on serial EMG), a temporary IA material is chosen [2]. These materials include saline, carboxymethylcellulose products (CMC) and Hyaluronic acid products (HA). Previous, but no longer available/clinically relevant short-term IA materials included gel foam, micronized acellular dermis and other collagen-based fillers, among others. Saline will not be discussed in detail; however, it is a reasonable choice when any augmentation could cause

© Springer Nature Singapore Pte Ltd. 2021
B.-J. Lee et al. (eds.), *Vocal Fold Injection*, https://doi.org/10.1007/978-981-16-3303-4_10

Table 10.1 Injection Augmentation Materials

Material	Average Duration of Effect (Range)
Non-hyaluronic acid	Short term
Saline	Hours
Carboxymethylcellulose (Renu gel, Prolaryn gel)	6 weeks (4–12 weeks)
Hyaluronic acid	
Restylane	12.2 weeks (3–6 months)
Juvederm	10.6 months (6–12 months)
Hylaform	6 months
Restylane Lyft (Perlane)	16.2 months (6–24 months)
	Durable/permanent
Calcium Hydroxylapatite	18 months (8–36 months)
Polydimethylsiloxane	Presumed permanent
Silk-hyaluronic acid	Potential for permanent

significant airway distress at the glottic level. The currently available short-term IA products will be discussed in detail.

In the setting of unilateral VF paralysis (permanent neurologic injury) without coexisting contralateral pathology contributing to glottic insufficiency, a durable, ideally permanent material is chosen for IA unilaterally into the affected VF. These materials include calcium hydroxylapatite products (CaHA), polydimethylsiloxane (PDMS) and silk-hyaluronic acid (Silk-HA). Previously used, but no longer available for durable IA, is polytetrafluoroethylene (Teflon) paste. The currently available long-term IA products will be discussed in detail.

Beyond the duration of benefit, the selection among injectables is influenced mostly by availability of the material (typically by country) and surgeon preference. CMC and HA products are both available in the United States (US), the European Union, and many other countries. However, in the US they require different processes for the surgeon to obtain them. HA products require a physician to order the chosen product directly from the company while CMC products can be purchased by a hospital or clinic as a medical implant otherwise would be. CaHA products are also widely available whereas PDMS is not available in the US. Silk-HA has only recently become available in the US. Surgeon preference for which VF augmentation material to choose is often based on prior positive or negative experience with a chosen material through personal patient outcomes and the ability to obtain and deliver their chosen material in the office or operating room (OR) setting (Table 10.1).

10.2 Short-Term Vocal Fold Injection Augmentation Materials

10.2.1 Carboxymethylcellulose Products

CMC products are the shortest acting of all off-the shelf IA materials and are ideal for short-term applications with a benefit of 4–12 weeks duration [1]. They are often used for a unilateral VF immobility when recovery is uncertain before the 6-month time point or when serial EMG has yet to show poor prognosis or synkinesis [2]. CMC products are also ideal in the setting when injection augmentation alone is unclear to help the patient's glottic insufficiency. For example, if there is an opposing motion abnormality, atrophy or scar, bilateral short-term augmentation may be chosen first as a diagnostic trial before durable augmentation is offered [3].

CMC products are sold under the names Prolaryn ™ Gel (Merz North America, Raleigh, NC, USA) and Renu® Gel (InHealth Technologies, Carpinteria, CA USA). Both products are a mixture of sodium CMC, glycerin and water. CMC products flow easily through a small gauge needle and can be delivered through any and all available injection approaches and devices. Both Prolaryn ™ Gel and Renu® Gel are FDA approved for vocal fold IA and have a track record of safety and efficacy [4].

10.2.2 Hyaluronic Acid Products

HA products have an intermediate duration of benefit between 3 and 12 months [5–9]. In its natural state HA is a naturally occurring extracellular matrix glycosaminoglycan found in various locations in the body, including the lamina propria of the VF. When HA is injected into the body, it binds with water and serves to fill out or "plump" the tissue into which it was injected. No HA product is FDA approved for use in vocal folds and is used "off label" for this indication. It is FDA approved as a dermal filler. While HA has similar rheologic properties to the lamina propria it does not prove effective for as a superficial, lamina propria VF filler [10, 11].

Because their duration of benefit is longer than 8 weeks, HA products can be used both for VF immobility of less than 6 months duration that is awaiting potential return of function and for longer-term applications. If used as a long-term augmentation material the patient must understand that the IA will need to be repeated. It is not the ideal choice for a patient who will need years of benefit.

The most common HA products in use are Restylane® (Galderma, Fort Worth, TX, USA), Juvederm® (Allergan, Irvine, CA, USA), Hylaform® Gel (Genzyme Biosurgery Inc., Ridgefield, NJ) and Restylane Lyft®, formerly Perlane® (Galderma, Fort Worth, TX, USA). The HA in these products is cross-linked to improve durability [12].

Juvederm® is longer acting than Restylane® due to a higher percentage of cross linking of the HA molecules that affords a thicker consistency [8]. Restylane® lasted 12.2 weeks on average in one study and up to 6 months in another [5, 7]. The clinical effect of Juvederm® lasted 10.6 months on average in a recent study [6]. Juvederm® is expected to more readily diffuse into tissue while Restylane® stays where it is placed. Restylane® performed well in a canine study that demonstrated superiority in injection localization compared to CMC on histological analysis [13].

Restylane® is made of biodegradable, non-animal stabilized HA generated by Streptococcus bacteria. It does not come from an animal source and thus is less likely to cause and allergic reaction. Inflammatory reactions, however, have been reported in 3.8% of VF IA in a recent publication [14]. It lasted 12.2 weeks on average in one study and up to 6 months in another [5, 7].

Hyalaform® is a modified HA product (Hylan B gel) derived from an avian source [9]. Those with allergies to avian proteins have the potential for reaction. Restylane Lyft® (Perlane®) has ten times the concentration and is longer lasting than Restylane® [7]. Restylane Lyft® was shown to maintain its effect on a group who only required one injection via EMG guidance at 16.2 months on average. In the same study a second group of patients required multiple injections with shorter intervals of improvement until ultimately satisfied. As is the case with any VF augmentation procedure in an immobile VF, reinnervation and natural muscle bulk can change over the course of the first year and may play a role in this study's outcomes [15].

10.3 Durable Vocal Fold Injection Augmentation Materials

10.3.1 Calcium Hydroxylapatite Products

CaHA has an average duration of benefit of 18 months (range 8–36 months) [16]. It is composed of Calcium hydroxyapatite microparticles in a CMC carrier. The particles are approximately 45 microns and can easily flow through a small gauge needle. The CMC carrier will be removed by the body at the same rate it would as a stand-alone short-term IA material, thus CaHA products are typically over-injected to anticipate this volume loss.

CaHA has a good safety profile [16, 17]. However, there are reports of inflammatory reactions and locoregional migration of the material [18]. In one canine study comparing Silk-HA to CaHA, CaHA was found outside the larynx and in one regional lymph node [19]. CaHA does not match well rheologically with native VF tissue, and thus it has the potential of changing more superficial vibration properties, even when placed correctly deep in the thyroarytenoid muscle [20].

The two available commercial CaHA products are Prolaryn™ Plus (Merz North America, Raleigh, NC, USA) and Renu® Voice (InHealth Technologies, Carpinteria, CA USA). They are both FDA approved for vocal fold IA. The two CaHA products are identical in composition, however the needles that are offered for OR and office per-oral IA are different. The Renu® needle has less tendency to clog during injection as compared to the Prolaryn™ product and the Renu® office per-oral/OR injection needle tip is longer compared to the one sold by Prolaryn™. The force needed to inject through the per-oral/OR injection needle is tolerable and does not typically require excessive pressure.

10.3.2 Polydimethylsiloxane

PDMS is presumed to be permanent [21]. It is a suspension of textured silicone particles with a mean diameter of 200 microns suspended in a polyvinylpyrrolidone hydrogel (PVP). It requires a large bore (i.e., 20 g) needle as supplied by the product manufacturer because particle size is not uniform and the particles can be as large as 500 microns [22, 23]. Due to its high viscosity, the amount of pressure needed to extrude the PDMS product can be significant [24].

The currently available PDMS product is the VOX® Implant (formerly Bioplastique ™, Laborie Medical, Geleen, The Netherlands). VOX® is sold with its own flexible catheter and a reusable injection administration device, akin to a caulking gun, to overcome the pressures needed to extrude the material.

VOX has a good safety profile overall [21]. However, there are case reports of significant inflammatory reactions requiring tracheotomy as well as foreign body reactions but no locoregional migration [25, 26]. VOX should be injected as far laterally, near/in the paraglottic space, as possible to avoid irregularities in the overlying epithelium. Because collagen replaces the PVP carrier with more volume than originally injected, over-injection of the material is not recommended [25].

10.3.3 Silk-Hyaluronic Acid

Silk-HA (Silk Voice®, Sofregen Medical, Medford, MA, USA) is a newer IA material that has just become available at the time of the writing of this chapter. Silk-HA is FDA approved for VF IA and is currently being used in a limited fashion and undergoing human safety and efficacy trials in the US.

Silk-HA has the potential for permanent medialization effect. It is composed of porous silk particles of 350–425 μm made from purified and liquified silk fibroin protein derived from the Bombyx mori silkworm that is freeze dried and mechanically made into particles. This process removes the immunogenic serocin coating affording no detectable immunogenicity on independent testing. The silk microparticles are suspended in a highly cross-linked hyaluronic acid [20].

Silk-HA demonstrated less stiffening of tissue in a porcine ex-vivo model as compared to CaHA. In 6 and 12-month canine histologic studies, collagen was found to be surrounding the still present Silk-HA material, slowly replacing the matrix with a fibrotic collagen matrix. Unlike PDMS where the silicone particles remain permanently, silk-HA is intended to be eventually removed and replaced with collagen to maintain its effect. In direct comparison to CaHA, Silk-HA was found outside the larynx in 1 animal and in no lymph nodes, while CaHA was found outside the larynx in 5 of 6 animals and in retropharyngeal lymph nodes in 2 of 6 animals [19, 27].

Silk is intended to be injected using a catheter delivery device through the working channel of a flexible laryngoscope in the awake patient. It can also be injected through a 23 g or larger needle in the OR or other routes in the office. Because it has the potential to be permanent, precision must be paramount when injecting the Silk-HA material. The catheter delivery device is designed to afford the user the ability to inject the material while maintaining precise control of the laryngoscope. An assistant remains necessary for in office use, although further catheter design innovation may 1 day make this truly a single operator procedure. To over inject, under inject or inject just the right amount is yet to be determined for Silk-HA.

Key Learning Points:

- Injection augmentation materials that are available "off–the-shelf" can be short acting or long acting/permanent.
- The choice of material is based on the potential for recovery of vocal fold motion, the patient's prognosis and the surgeon's preference (what materials are available to the surgeon and what the surgeon feels comfortable injecting in the office or operating room settings).
- Short acting injection materials (typically saline or carboxymethylcellulose) can be used in a diagnostic fashion when it is unclear if injection augmentation alone will improve a patient's symptoms or if unilateral or bilateral augmentation is in question due to other glottic pathology or airway concerns.
- Short acting materials include carboxymethylcellulose products (4–8 weeks duration) and hyaluronic acid products (3–12 months duration).
- Durable materials include calcium hydroxylapatite products (18 months duration on average), polydimethylsiloxane (presumed permanent) and silk-hyaluronic acid (potential for permanent effect).

References

1. Mallur PS, Rosen CA. Vocal fold injection: review of indications, techniques, and materials for augmentation. Clin Exp Otorhinolaryngol. 2010;3(4):177–82.
2. Munin MC, Rosen CA, Zullo T. Utility of laryngeal electromyography in predicting recovery after vocal fold paralysis. Arch Phys Med Rehabil. 2003;84(8):1150–3.
3. Carroll TL, Rosen CA. Trial vocal fold injection. J Voice. 2010;24(4):494–8.
4. Mallur PS, Morrison MP, Postma GN, Amin MR, Rosen CA. Safety and efficacy of carboxymethylcellulose in the treatment of glottic insufficiency. Laryngoscope. 2012;122(2):322–6.
5. Halderman AA, Bryson PC, Benninger MS, Chota R. Safety and length of benefit of Restylane for office-based injection medialization—a retrospective review of one Institution's experience. J Voice. 2014;28(5):631–5.
6. Bertroche JT, Radder M, Kallogjeri D, Paniello RC, Bradley JP. Patient-defined duration of benefit from juvederm (hyaluronic acid) used in injection laryngoplasty. Laryngoscope. 2019;129(12):2744–7.
7. Lau DP, Lee GA, Wong SM, Lim VP, Chan YH, Tan NG, et al. Injection Laryngoplasty with hyaluronic acid for unilateral vocal cord paralysis. Randomized controlled trial comparing two different particle sizes. J Voice. 2010;24(1):113–8.
8. Gutowski KA. Hyaluronic acid fillers. Clin Plast Surg. 2016;43(3):489–96.
9. Hertegard S, Hallen L, Laurent C, Lindstrom E, Olofsson K, Testad P, et al. Cross-linked hyaluronan versus collagen for injection treatment of glottal insufficiency: 2-year follow-up. Acta Otolaryngol. 2004;124(10):1208–14.
10. Caton T, Thibeault SL, Klemuk S, Smith ME. Viscoelasticity of Hyaluronan and Nonhyaluronan based vocal fold Injectables: implications for mucosal versus muscle use. Laryngoscope. 2007;117(3):516–21.
11. Kimura M, Mau T, Chan RW. Viscoelastic properties of phonosurgical biomaterials at phonatory frequencies. Laryngoscope. 2010;120(4):764–8.
12. Salinas JB, Chhetri DK. Injection Laryngoplasty: techniques and choices of fillers. Curr Otorhinolaryngol Rep. 2014;2(2):131–6.
13. Zeitels SM, Lombardo PJ, Chaves JL, Faquin WC, Hillman RE, Heaton JT, et al. Vocal fold injection of absorbable materials: a histologic analysis with clinical ramifications. Ann Otol Rhinol Laryngol. 2019;128(3_suppl):71S–81S.
14. Dominguez LM, Tibbetts KM, Simpson CB. Inflammatory reaction to hyaluronic acid: a newly described complication in vocal fold augmentation: inflammatory reaction to HA. Laryngoscope. 2017;127(2):445–9.
15. Wang C-C, Chang M-H, Jiang R-S, Lai H-C, Virgilio AD, Wang C-P, et al. Laryngeal electromyography-guided hyaluronic acid vocal fold injection for unilateral vocal fold paralysis: a prospective long-term follow-up outcome report. JAMA Otolaryngol Head Neck Surg. 2015;141(3):264–71.
16. Carroll TL, Rosen CA. Long-term results of calcium hydroxylapatite for vocal fold augmentation. Laryngoscope. 2011;121(2):313–9.
17. Lee M, Lee DY, Kwon T-K. Safety of office-based percutaneous injection laryngoplasty with calcium hydroxylapatite. Laryngoscope. 2019;129(10):2361–5.
18. Tanna N, Zalkind D, Glade RS, Bielamowicz SA. Foreign body reaction to calcium Hydroxylapatite vocal fold augmentation. Arch Otolaryngol Head Neck Surg. 2006;132(12):1379–82.

19. Gulka CP, Brown JE, Giordano JEM, Hickey JE, Montero MP, Hoang A, et al. A novel silk-based vocal fold augmentation material: 6-month evaluation in a canine model. Laryngoscope. 2019;129(8):1856–62.
20. Brown JE, Gulka CP, Giordano JEM, Montero MP, Hoang A, Carroll TL. Injectable silk protein microparticle-based fillers: a novel material for potential use in Glottic insufficiency. J Voice. 2019;33(5):773–80.
21. Mattioli F, Bettini M, Botti C, Busi G, Tassi S, Malagoli A, et al. Polydimethylsiloxane injection laryngoplasty for unilateral vocal fold paralysis: long-term results. J Voice. 2017;31(4):517.e1–517.e7.
22. Hagemann M, Seifert E. The use of polydimethylsiloxane for injection Laryngoplasty. World J Surg. 2008;32(9):1940–7.
23. Sittel C, Echtemach M, Federspil PA, Plinkert PK. Polydimethylsiloxane particles for permanent injection Laryngoplasty. Ann Otol Rhinol Laryngol. 2006;115(2):103–9.
24. Sittel C. Larynx: implants and stents. GMS Curr Top Otorhinolaryngol Head Neck Surg [Internet]. 2011 Mar 10 [cited 2020 Sep 7];8. https://www.ncbi.nlm.nih.gov/pmc/articles/PMC3199813/
25. Randhawa PS, Ramsay AD, Rubin JS. Foreign body reaction to polymethylsiloxane gel (Bioplastique™) after vocal fold augmentation. J Laryngol Otol. 2008;122(7):750–3.
26. Ovari A, Witt G, Schuldt T, Hingst V, Pau H-W, Jäckel M, et al. Polydimethylsiloxane for injection laryngoplasty: two cases necessitating tracheotomy. Eur Arch Otorhinolaryngol. 2014;271(4):839–44.
27. Carroll TL. A novel silk based vocal fold augmentation material: 12-month evaluation in a Canine Model. October 2018. Paper presented at the fall voice conference, Seattle, WA.

Autologous Materials for Vocal Fold Augmentation

11

Byung-Joo Lee

Abstract

Various materials can be used for injection laryngoplasty. Autologous materials are immunologically safe compared to other non-autologous materials, so they do not cause foreign body reactions or chronic inflammation. However, there is a disadvantage that it requires general anesthesia compared to commercialized products. The autologous materials currently used in clinical practice are fat and cartilage. Fat has an advantage because it has excellent viscoelasticity, but it has a disadvantage of having resorption. There is a disadvantage in that it is difficult to predict the clinical outcome after fat injection due to various resorption rates. Cartilage is not a popular method, but it has the advantage of lasting long-term effects with a single injection.

Keywords

Autologous injection material · Fat · Cartilage

B.-J. Lee (✉)
Department of Otorhinolaryngology,
Pusan National University Hospital,
Pusan, Korea (Republic of)

11.1 Introduction

Glottis insufficiency causes dysphonia, which significantly reduces the patient's quality of life. There are several varieties of surgical methods and nonsurgical methods to improve glottis contact [1]. Laryngeal frame surgery, such as thyroplasty or arytenoid adduction, is a good surgical method. However, such open surgery has the disadvantage of creating scars on the neck. Therefore, injection laryngoplasty has been widely practiced recently. When performing injection laryngoplasty, it can be divided into various techniques according to the injection route, and there are advantages and disadvantages for each route [2, 3]. It can also be classified according to the type of filler material used in injection laryngoplasty. Filler types can be classified according to duration. Also, it can be classified into autologous or non-autologous according to the source of the filler. The various types of fillers and their pros and cons were explained in the previous chapter. This chapter focuses on autologous fat and autologous cartilage used as autologous vocal fold injection materials.

11.2 Autologous Fat Injection

11.2.1 Introduction

Autologous fat injection was first developed in early 1990 and widely used because of many

© Springer Nature Singapore Pte Ltd. 2021
B.-J. Lee et al. (eds.), *Vocal Fold Injection*, https://doi.org/10.1007/978-981-16-3303-4_11

merits over other injection materials including that, above all, it has no worry of tissue rejection due to its autologous nature, usually abundant in amount from many donor sites and excellent viscoelastic properties similar to the vocal folds [4]. The downside of fat includes that it requires a donor site but most critical downside is difficult to predict the amount of resorption in the recipient site. An animal study reported up to 82% resorption in amount 12 weeks after the vocal fold injection, 68% of those injected with fat and insulin, and 71% in those combined with thyroplasty [5]. Shindo et al. reported the follow-up result from 12 patients injected with autologous fat for 1 year that shows the best result in 2 months after the injection and then stabilizes 6 months after the injection [6]. The resorption amount varies 20–60% among studies [7, 8].

There no question that once survives in the vocal fold, the autologous fat is the most ideal injectable. Although there have been multiple trial to increase survival of the fat graft, there is no single method is superior. But it is well accepted that great care should be taken in fat harvest because the fatty acid, blood cells components produced by fat harvest procedure are strong inflammation mediators and can induce edema and breathing problem when injected into the vocal folds. Therefore, fat harvest should be done with a large bore needle and a low pressure aspiration to minimize fat cell destruction. And also a washing process after fat harvest is imperative. The author adopted a low pressure fat aspiration and purified by centrifugation. There are many other fat tissue treatment including washing, gravity separation, and filtration, but there is no single standardized technique for fat tissue processing [9].

11.2.2 Surgical Techniques

Fat tissue has excellent viscoelasticity but it can significantly hamper the vocal fold vibration if injected in the superficial layer of the vocal fold. In fat injection procedure, a large bore injection needle is used to avoid fat cell destruction. With this large bore needle (usually 19 gauge), it is difficult to control the depth of injection, so injection should be aimed to the deep muscular area or paraglottic space away from the free edge of the vocal fold.

Lipoinjection needs a specialized device called Bruening syringe, which has a ratchet mechanism that enables the surgeon to inject a controlled amount of fat with less effort (Fig. 11.1).

11.2.2.1 Liposuction

Under general anesthesia, the abdomen is disinfected and draped properly to expose lower abdomen above the anterior superior iliac spine. The whole fat harvest procedure should be aseptic.

First, the skin infiltration with 1:100,000 epinephrine and 2% lidocaine mixture at the inner side of the umbilicus on the side of fat harvest. Skin incision less than 1 cm along inner side of the umbilicus to avoid external scar. Subcutaneous tissue is dissected with mosquito until the fat layer appears. About 60 cc of tumescent solution is injected widely over the area where the fat is to be aspirated. A tumescent solution contains lidocaine, epinephrine and large amount of Ringer's lactate solution and provide bloodless fat aspiration.

After 20 minutes, a 6 mm liposuction cannula is connected with 10–20 cm^3 syringe and the tip of the cannula is inserted through the skin incision, then pull the plunge to make a negative

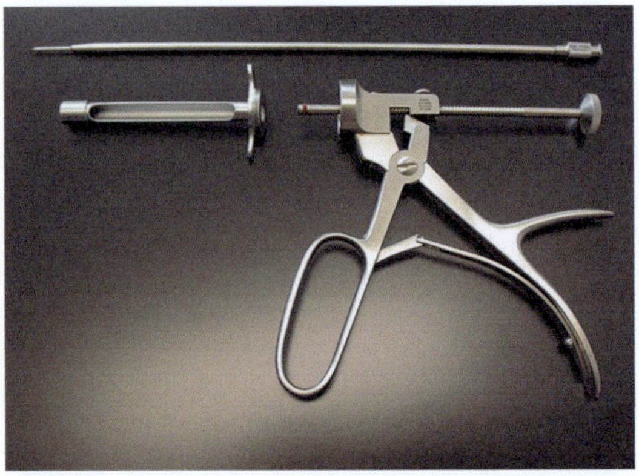

Fig. 11.1 Bruening syringe. This is also called Arnold-Bruening syringe that has a ratchet system to deliver the fat into the vocal fold with controlled amount. Each audible click ejects about 0.2 cm^3 of fat

pressure and start moving the cannula back and forth around the subcutaneous layer observing crushed fat tissue is aspirated into the syringe (Fig. 11.2). Maintaining a negative pressure in the syringe during whole aspiration procedure is important for a successful result. For a hand-held syringe, a towel clip can be used to anchor the plunger in place (Fig. 11.3). After fat aspiration, the skin incision is loosely closed with one stitch of nylon suture and a compressive dressing done around the abdomen.

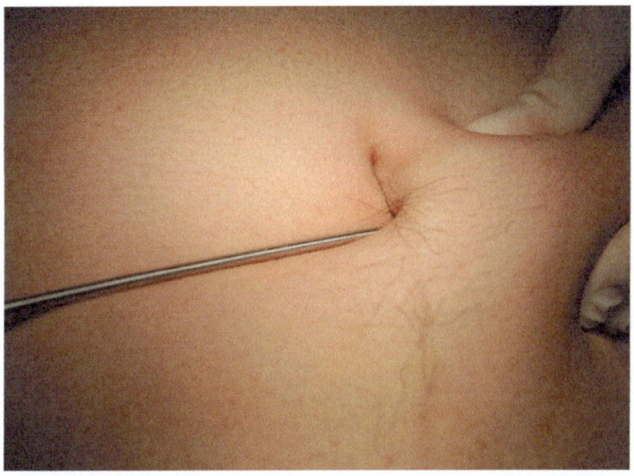

Fig. 11.2 Cannula insertion and fat aspiration. After making small incision along inner side of the umbilicus and dissection subcutaneous tissue with Mosquitos, a 6 mm cannula is inserted into the subcutaneous fat layer

11.2.2.2 Fat Purification

Aspirates is transferred to containers and centrifuged at 4000 rpm for 1 min. The fat aspirates is divided in to three layers: a top layer of oil from destroyed fat cells, a middle layer of viable fat cells and a bottom layer of blood and cell debris (Fig. 11.4). The bottom fluid is drained and the top oil layer is carefully removed using cotton tip leaving usable fat layer. Then the fat layer is gently transferred to the 1 cm^3 syringe using two-way connector (Fig. 11.5).

11.2.2.3 Fat Injection

The Bruening syringe is assembled and the syringe with fat is loaded. The plunger of the Bruening syringe is carefully inserted into the fat syringe and the needle is primed with small amount of fat. Care should be taken to keep the needle tip aseptic.

Then the drape is changed for microlaryngeal surgery. A suspension laryngoscope is inserted as usual microscopic surgery and the target vocal fold is exposed. Zero degree rigid long laryngeal endoscope with camera provides better exposure than laryngeal microscopy because the handle of the Bruening syringe blocks the surgeon's view when used with microscopy.

With endoscopic guidance, the needle tip is inserted lateral to the arcuate line deep into

Fig. 11.3 The fat aspiration syringe locked with towel clips. This locking system maintains a negative pressure inside the syringe during fat aspiration procedure

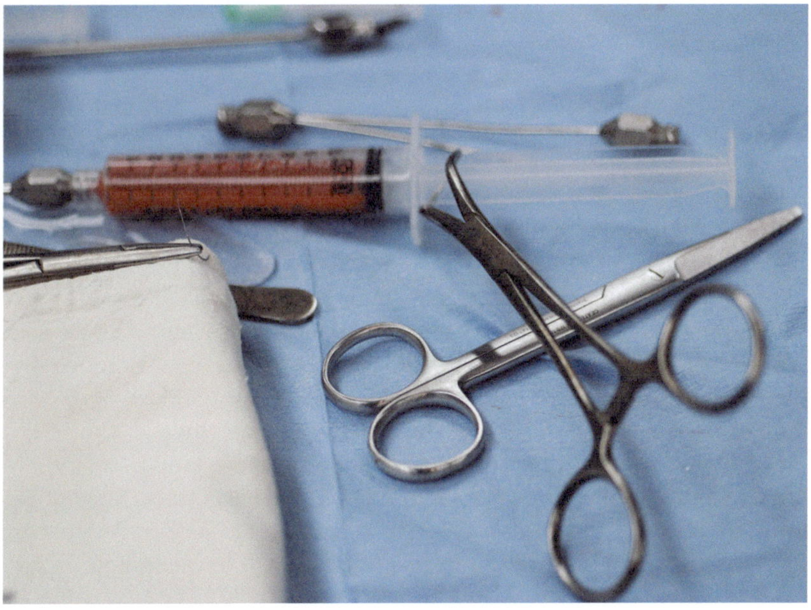

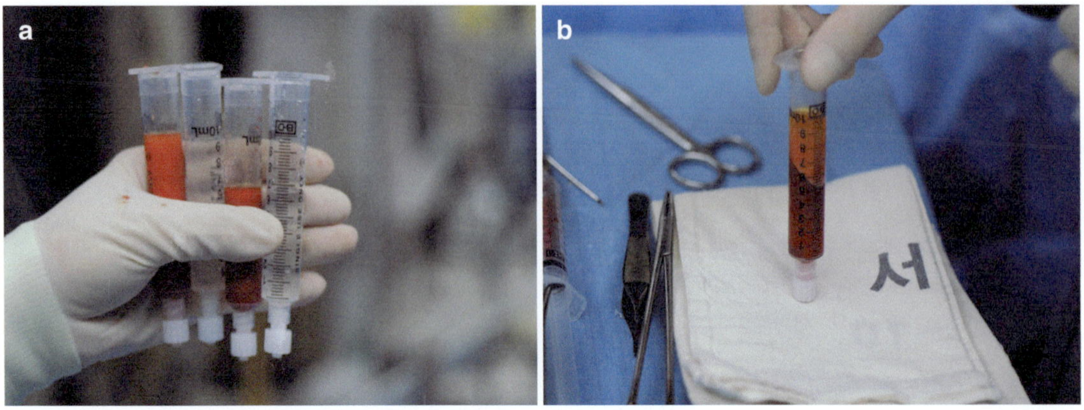

Fig. 11.4 Fat aspirates purification by the centrifugation. (**a**). Fat aspirates right after the aspiration. (**b**). Fat aspirates forms 3 layers after 1 min of 4000 rpm centrifugation

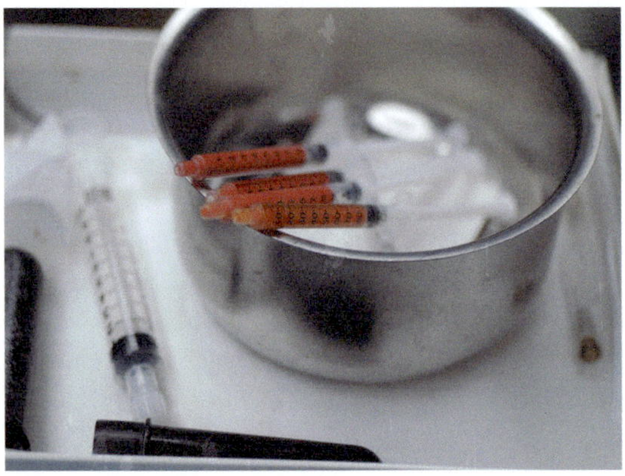

Fig. 11.5 The fat transferred to the 1 cc syringes for the injection. Fat was transferred to 1 cc syringe using 2 ways connector. Care must be taken not to apply too much pressure to avoid fat cell destruction

the thyroarytenoid muscle or paraglottic fat space (Fig. 11.6a). Once the needle penetrates the vocal fold mucosa, it is moved a little to the lateral direction and then advanced into the muscle layer. By doing this technique, the needle leaves a zigzag path that seals the needle track preventing retrograde spillage of fat. For the paralyzed vocal fold, the injection is directed to the lateral aspect of the vocal process of the arytenoid cartilage, then additional injection can be done in the mid-portion of the vocal fold. The amount of injection varies according to the size of the larynx, but about 50% overinjection is recommended considering resorption (Fig. 11.6b).

11.2.3 Advantage and Disadvantage

The advantage of fat as an injection material is that it is very similar to the viscoelasticity of the vocal folds compared to other materials. And fat has the advantage of being easily obtained by a simple procedure. However, the injected fat is resorbed, and the degree of resorption is difficult to predict. So, repeated fat injection may be necessary. And, general anesthesia is required to inject autologous fat.

11.3 Autologous Cartilage Injection

11.3.1 Introduction

Cartilage graft is one of most popular volumetric material that is widely used in plastic surgery and reconstructive surgeries, such as rhinoplasty or otoplasty [10, 11]. The transplantation of autologous cartilage has low extrusion rates, low blood supply requirements, and high survival rates. So, autologous cartilage graft is safe because there is no foreign body reaction after transplantation. In addition, the viability of the

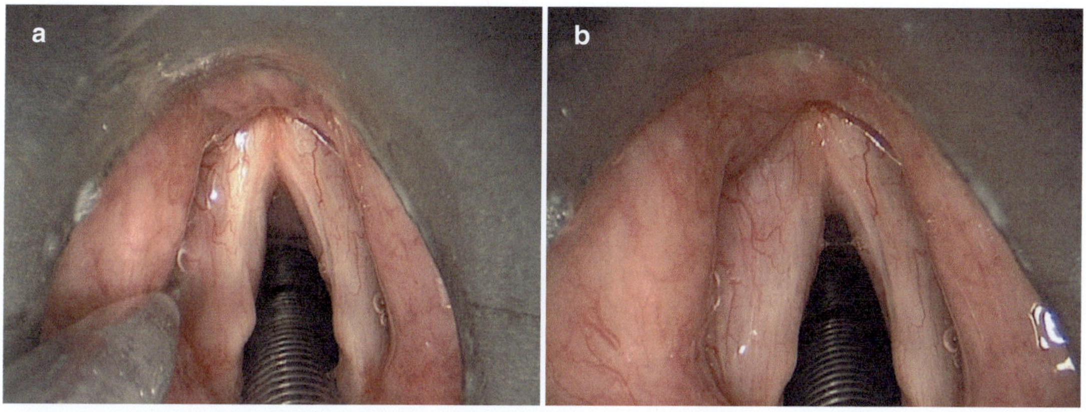

Fig. 11.6 Fat injection on the vocal fold. A long rigid endoscope provides better view than a microscope. (**a**). The needle is inserted lateral to the arcuate line of the vocal fold. (**b**). Increase volume of the vocal fold after fat injection

grafted cartilage is lost, but the overall volume is maintained for a long time [12, 13]. In a study in which thyroplasty was performed using thyroid alar or auricular elastic cartilage as graft material, the overall volume of grafted cartilage was maintained over 85% even after 6 months of transplantation [14, 15].

The study using cartilage as a material for vocal fold augmentation was published in 1955 by Arnold [16]. Harvested cartilage from rib or nasal septum was injected into the vocal cords using procaine-penicillin oil as a vehicle, but foreign body reactions occurred due to the injected oil. Lee et al. minced the harvested auricular cartilage with a knife and scissor and injected it into the vocal folds using autologous fat as a vehicle. The autologous cartilage injected into the vocal folds lost the viability of chondrocytes, but remained well within the vocal folds for 3 years without any foreign body reaction or inflammatory reaction [12, 13].

11.3.2 Surgical Technique and Clinical Outcome (Fig. 11.7)

The laryngeal exposure should be evaluated before performing the surgery. Under general anesthesia, cartilage and fat are harvested from the auricle and abdomen, respectively. Auricular cartilage is harvested through posterior auricular vertical incision. Harvested auricular cartilage is minced small enough to pass through a 19 gauze needle using a blade and a scissor. Abdominal fat is used as a vehicle for injecting cartilage. Abdominal fat is harvested through peri-umbrical incision. Harvest fat is cut finely using a scalpel and a scissor. After filling the minced cartilage and fat into a 1 ml syringe, inject the minced cartilage using a Bruening injector. Minced cartilage is injected into vocalis muscle at the junction of the middle and posterior third of the vocal fold under laryngeal microscope with the slope of the Bruening injector needle made to face outside. Care should be taken as superficial injection can lead to permanent dysphonia. Also, a little leak may occur to the site where the injected cartilage was injected. In general, about 0.5 ml of cartilage is injected, but the amount varies depending on the individual for optimal consequences.

Since intracordal cartilage injection is not yet a popular method in the area of injection laryngoplasty, there is one report on clinical outcome. Lim et al. reported the results of injection laryngoplasty using autologous minced cartilage in 29 patients with vocal cord paralysis [17]. Perceptual assessments by GRBAS scale, acoustic parameters of jitter, shimmer, noise-to-harmonic ratio, and maximum phonation time were significantly

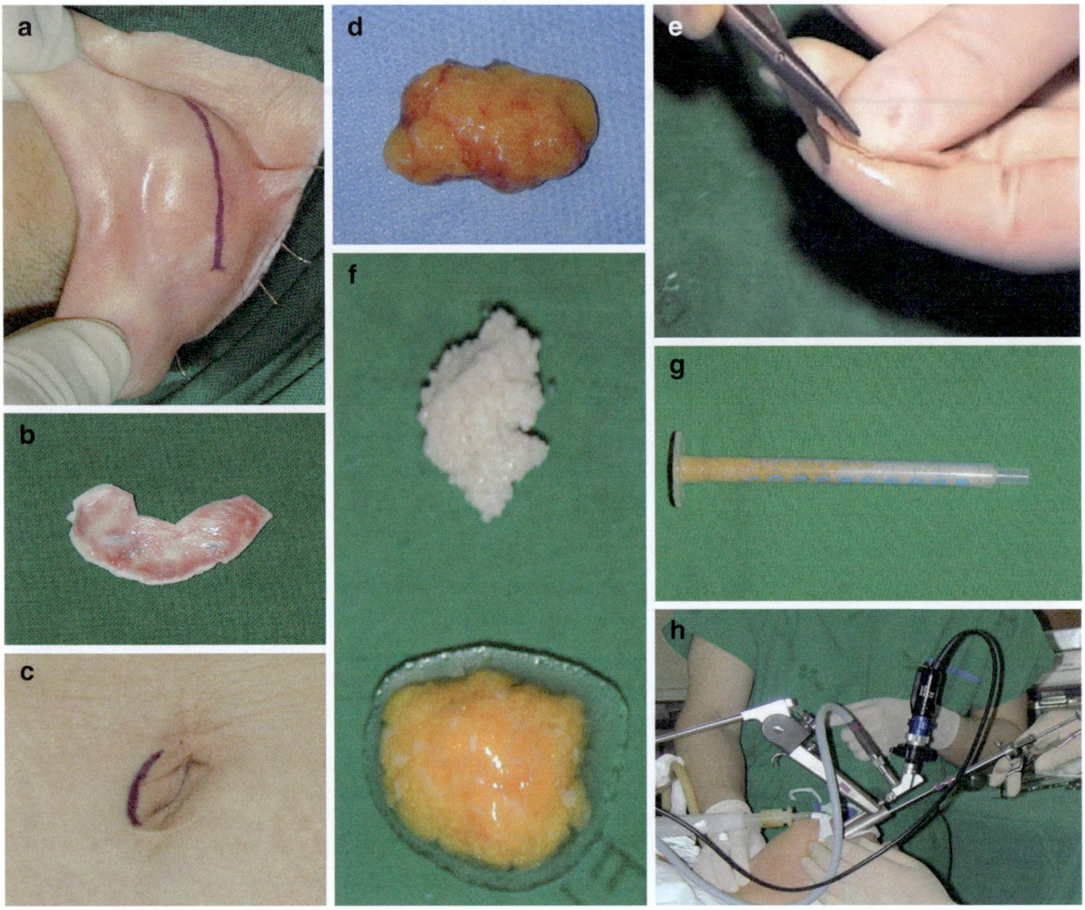

Fig. 11.7 Surgical procedure of injection laryngoplasty using minced autologous cartilage and fat. Under general anesthesia, auricular cartilage is harvested through posterior auricular incision (**a**, **b**). Fat is harvested through periumbrical incision (**c**, **d**). Using a knife and scissor (**e**), chop the harvested cartilage (white color) and fat (yellow color) (**f**). After filling the syringe with chopped cartilage (white color) and fat (yellow color), it is injected into the vocal cords under a rigid laryngoscope (**g**, **h**)

improved even after one injection 12 months after injection. And no significant complications such as foreign body reaction, granuloma formation, or inflammation were observed.

11.3.3 Advantage and Disadvantage

The advantage of injection laryngoplasty using minced autologous cartilage is that the volume is maintained for a long time due to the characteristics of cartilage without foreign body reaction. So, in patients with vocal cord paralysis, even with a single injection, there is an improvement in the voice for more than a year [17].

The disadvantage of autologous intracordal cartilage injection is that general anesthesia is required. Then, the harvested cartilage and fat must be chopped in order to pass through the 19-gauge needle. This process is time-consuming. In order to overcome these limitations, the quick and easy way to make cartilage flakes using the freezing and grinding technique was introduced [18]. In addition, there are studies to use decellularized allogenic or xenogenic cartilage to overcome the disadvantages using autologous cartilage [19–21].

Key Learning Points:

- There are fat and cartilage as autologous materials that can be used for injection laryngoplasty.
- Fat has good viscoelasticity, but has the disadvantage of being absorbed. It is difficult to predict the result due to various resorption rates.
- Cartilage has the advantage of lasting a long time with a single injection. It is not a popular method yet, but it is thought to be a promising method.

References

1. Siu J, Tam S, Fung K. A comparison of outcomes in interventions for unilateral vocal fold paralysis: a systematic review. Laryngoscope. 2016;126(7):1616–24.
2. Mallur PS, Rosen CA. Vocal fold injection: review of indications, techniques, and materials for augmentation. Clin Exp Otorhinolaryngol. 2010;3(4):177–82.
3. Sulica L, Rosen CA, Postma GN, Simpson B, Amin M, Courey M, et al. Current practice in injection augmentation of the vocal folds: indications, treatment principles, techniques, and complications. Laryngoscope. 2010;120(2):319–25.
4. Chan RW, Titze IR. Viscosities of implantable biomaterials in vocal fold augmentation surgery. Laryngoscope. 1998;108(5):725–31.
5. Kruschewsky Lde S, de Mello-Filho FV, dos Santos AC, Rosen CA. Autologous fat graft absorption in unilateral paralyzed canine vocal folds. Laryngoscope. 2007;117(1):96–100.
6. Shindo ML, Zaretsky LS, Rice DH. Autologous fat injection for unilateral vocal fold paralysis. Ann Otol Rhinol Laryngol. 1996;105(8):602–6.
7. Laccourreye O, Hans S, Ménard M, Hacquart N, Brasnu D, Crevier-Buchman L. Results of intracordal injection of autologous fat in postoperative laryngeal paralysis. Chirurgie. 1999;124(3):283–7.
8. McCulloch TM, Andrews BT, Hoffman HT, Graham SM, Karnell MP, Minnick C. Long-term follow-up of fat injection laryngoplasty for unilateral vocal cord paralysis. Laryngoscope. 2002;112(7 Pt 1):1235–8.
9. Truzzi GM, Pauna HF, Bette P, Gusmão RJ, Crespo AN, Semenzati GO. Methods of fat tissue processing for human vocal fold injection: a systematic review. J Voice. 2017;31(2):244.e17-.e21.
10. Liang X, Wang K, Malay S, Chung KC, Ma J. A systematic review and meta-analysis of comparison between autologous costal cartilage and alloplastic materials in rhinoplasty. J Plast Reconstr Aesthet Surg. 2018;71(8):1164–73.
11. Okajima H, Suzuki K, Takeichi Y, Umeda K, Baba S. Long-term results of otoplasty for microtia. Acta Otolaryngol Suppl. 1996;525:25–9.
12. Lee BJ, Wang SG, Goh EK, Chon KM, Lee CH. Intracordal injection of autologous auricular cartilage in the paralyzed canine vocal fold. Otolaryngol Head Neck Surg. 2004;131(1):34–43.
13. Lee BJ, Wang SG, Goh EK, Chon KM, Lee CH, Lorenz RR. Histologic evaluation of intracordal autologous cartilage injection in the paralyzed canine vocal fold at two and three years. Otolaryngol Head Neck Surg. 2006;134(4):627–30.
14. Guay ME, Miller FR, Bauer TW, Tucker HM. Vocal fold medialization using autologous cartilage in a canine model: a preliminary study. Laryngoscope. 1995;105(10):1049–52.
15. Caballero M, Bernal-Sprekelsen M, Farré X, Calvo C, Alós L. Autologous elastic cartilage for laryngoplasty: histologic evaluation in a rabbit model. Ann Otol Rhinol Laryngol. 2003;112(8):734–9.
16. Arnold GE. [Injection of new substances with the Brüning syringe in correction of unilateral recurrent nerve paralysis]. Arch Ohren Nasen Kehlkopfheilkd. 1955;167(2–6):508–10; discussion, 19–21.
17. Lim YS, Lee YS, Lee JC, Lee BJ, Wang SG, Park HJ, et al. Intracordal auricular cartilage injection for unilateral vocal fold paralysis. J Biomed Mater Res B Appl Biomater. 2015;103(1):47–51.
18. Park YM, Lee WY, Lim YS, Lee JC, Lee BJ, Wang SG. New technique for preparing cartilage for intracordal injection: the freezing and grinding method. J Voice. 2014;28(4):508–11.
19. Lee JC, Lee BJ, Wang SG, Lee CH, Shin DH. Intracordal injections with allogenic cartilage in a canine paralyzed vocal fold model: long-term results. J Voice. 2012;26(4):515–20.
20. Kang DW, Shin SC, Jang JY, Park HY, Lee JC, Wang SG, et al. Decellularization of human nasal septal cartilage for the novel filler material of vocal fold augmentation. J Voice. 2017;31(1):127.e1-.e6.
21. Shin SC, Park HY, Shin N, Jung DW, Kwon HK, Kim JM, et al. Evaluation of decellularized xenogenic porcine auricular cartilage as a novel biocompatible filler. J Biomed Mater Res B Appl Biomater. 2018;106(7):2708–15.

EMG Guided Injection Laryngoplasty

12

Chen-Chi Wang

Abstract

Laryngeal electromyography (EMG) is the only test that can provide laryngologists with the neuromuscular status and prognostic information of patients with unilateral vocal fold paralysis (UVFP). Compared to normal side vocal fold, the paralyzed thyroarytenoid/lateral cricoarytenoid (TA/LCA) muscle complex usually show characteristic signals on laryngeal EMG such as fibrillation signal when the patient keep silent; or reduced recruitment of motor unit potentials when the patient phonate vowel/i/. By using a 25–26 gauge monopolar injectable needle electrode, 1 ml of commercially available forgiving filler such as hyaluronic acid could be delivered into the TA/LCA muscle complex of paralyzed vocal fold via the transcervical cricothyroid membrane puncture under laryngeal EMG guidance. The injection augmentation could be done when the patient is in a relatively stable and comfortable supine position without the need of laryngoscopy. The injection augmentation effect may last long term and open surgery could be avoided. If patients experienced symptoms recurrence after absorption of fillers, prognostic information obtained from laryngeal EMG could be used to guide further management such as repeated injection for patients with good prognosis or prompt thyroplasty type I for patients with poor prognosis. It is an ideal initial management for patients of UVFP.

Keywords

Electromyography · Hyaluronic acid Injection laryngoplasty · Thyroarytenoid muscle · Lateral cricoarytenoid muscle Cricothyroid membrane · Spontaneous activity · Fibrillation · Recruitment · Motor unit potential

12.1 Unilateral Vocal Fold Paralysis

Unilateral vocal fold paralysis (UVFP) is a common disorder in the practice of otolaryngology. Incomplete vocal fold adduction in UVFP may cause formation of a constant glottal gap, which is usually associated with breathy voice and aspiration during swallowing. The impairment of recurrent laryngeal nerve function can have various causes, but idiopathic and iatrogenic types are the most frequent conditions [1, 2]. For

C.-C. Wang (✉)
Department of Otorhinolaryngology-Head & Neck Surgery, Taichung Veterans General Hospital, Taichung, Taiwan

School of Medicine, National Yang Ming Chiao Tung University, Taipei, Taiwan

Department of Audiology and Speech-Language Pathology, Asia University, Taichung, Taiwan

© Springer Nature Singapore Pte Ltd. 2021
B.-J. Lee et al. (eds.), *Vocal Fold Injection*, https://doi.org/10.1007/978-981-16-3303-4_12

patients with UVFP, four types of surgical interventions are available for correction of the glottal gap [3]. Three of them are open surgeries including medialization thyroplasty (or thyroplasty type I), ayrtenoid adduction, and laryngeal reinnervation which are usually reserved for patients with persistent UVFP. The injection laryngoplasty is a minimal invasive management that is usually chosen in the early stage of UVFP. For patients with UVFP, knowing their disease prognosis and then deciding a proper management for rehabilitation of laryngeal function are very important.

12.2 Laryngeal EMG

Laryngeal electromyography (EMG) was introduced in 1944 by Weddel and Pattle, [4] and advanced substantially in the 1950s by Faaborg-Andersen, [5] Buchthal, [6] and others. However, European Laryngological Society noted that although laryngeal EMG has been considered as a valuable diagnostic tool for more than several decades, many laryngologists do not routinely use it [7]. In fact, USA study group indicated that laryngeal EMG is an invaluable adjunct to laryngologic assessment. It is easy to perform, well-tolerated, and presents minimal risks to patients [8]. Specifically, laryngeal EMG is the only test that can provide laryngologists with the neuromuscular status of UVFP patients. Therefore, it is essential for a modern laryngologist to obtain the basic knowledge and techniques of laryngeal EMG.

12.2.1 Basic Neurophysiology of Larynx

The interior of a muscle or nerve cell is electrically negative with respect to its exterior. The electrical potential difference is called the resting membrane potential. The resting membrane potential reflects the ionic gradient of the cell membrane. The intracellular compartment has a high concentration of potassium and the extracellular compartment has a high concentration of sodium and chloride. The gradient is maintained by active transport over the cell membrane. With the application of an appropriate stimulus, nerves and muscles generate action potential. Action potential is a fast and transient reversal of the membrane potential caused by a temporary change in cell membrane permeability [8].

The motor unit consists of the cell body and axon of a single lower motor neuron, the neuromuscular junction, and all the muscle fibers the motor neuron innervates. The motor neuron transmits electrical signals that cause muscles to contract. An EMG uses electrodes to record the electrical signals which could be used to evaluate the health of motor unit (Fig. 12.1). It also helps differentiate the dysfunction site of nerve, neuromuscular junction or muscle. In larynx, the intrinsic laryngeal muscles are responsible for controlling voice production. The intrinsic laryngeal muscles are controlled by superior and inferior (recurrent) laryngeal nerves branching from tenth cranial nerve, vagus nerve. Except circothyroid (CT) muscle that is innervated by superior laryngeal nerve (SLN), all other intrinsic laryngeal muscles including thyroarytenoid (TA) muscle, lateral cricoarytenoid (LCA) muscle, interarytenoid (IA) muscle and posterior cricoarytenoid muscles (PCA) are controlled by recurrent laryngeal nerve (RLN) and are responsible for adduction and abduction of vocal folds. Impairment of RLN function could induce vocal fold paralysis. The EMG signal obtained from TA/LCA complex therefore could be used for diagnosing the function of RLN.

12.2.2 The Electrodiagnostic Apparatus

In most EMG laboratories, sophisticated, multichannel systems are used with the advantages of permitting simultaneous, multichannel recording. There are several excellent systems available commercially. However, EMG is usually not a standard equipment in many otolaryngological departments. A cost-effective option for otolaryngolotists is the use of the Auditory Brain-stem Response (ABR) audiometer found in many offices. However, they should be used in addition to, not in place of, a sophisticated EMG system

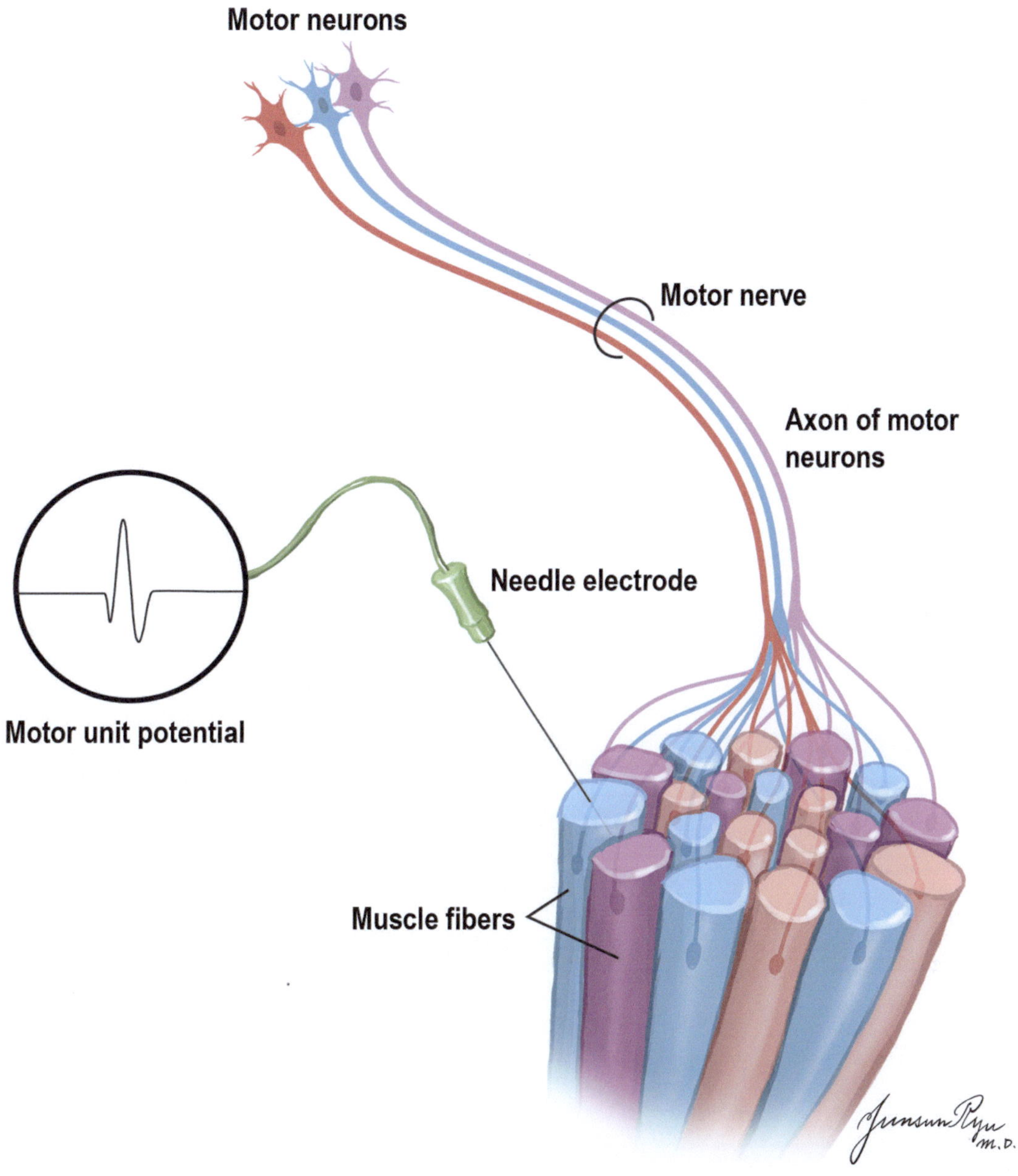

Fig. 12.1 EMG uses an electrode to record the electrical signals (such as motor unit potential) transmitted from a single motor neuron to cause contraction of muscle fibers the neuron innervates

for diagnosing testing [8]. Therefore, cooperation with experienced neurologist and using the facility in neurologic department are highly recommended. For otolaryngologists, quick familiar with EMG technique could be achieved through mutual discussion with experienced neurologists. The neurologist could help record and interpret the data while otolaryngologists focus on vocal fold puncture and EMG guided injection management which will be described in later paragraphs.

The electrical signals generated in the motor unit could be recorded by electrodes, which include surface or needle electrodes. Surface electrodes are noninvasive and are placed on the skin or mucosa. But they are the least selective electrode type and are not suitable for recording details of individual laryngeal muscles. There are several types of needle electrodes: monopolar, bipolar, concentric, single fiber, and hooked wire [9] (Fig. 12.2). The monopolar needle electrode is a solid stainless steel needle that is insulated except at its tip. Working with the reference elec-

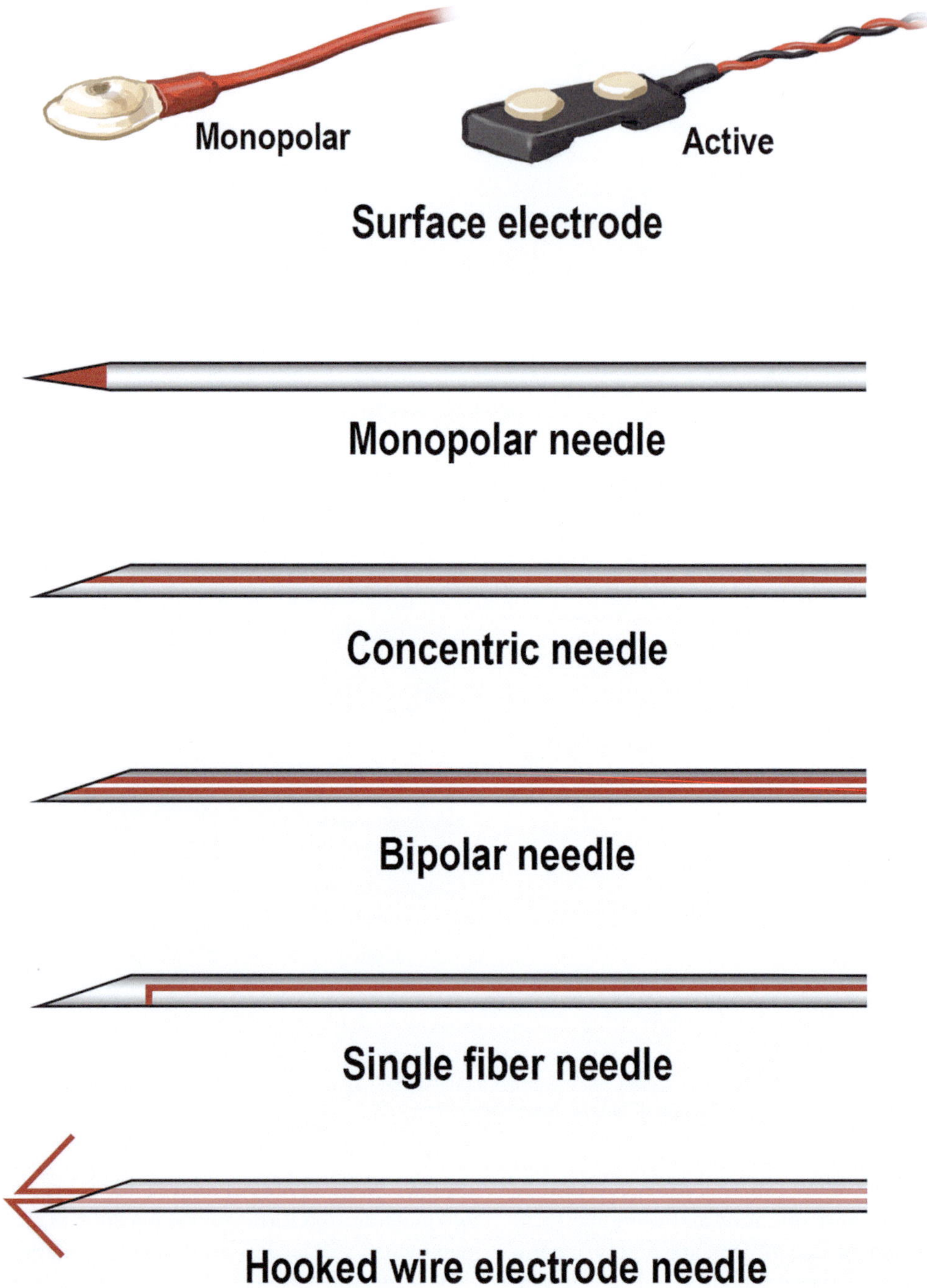

Fig. 12.2 Different types of EMG electrodes. (Redrawn based on the chapter "The EMG as a window to the brain: signal processing tools to enhance the view" in the book "Advances in Processing and Pattern Analysis of Biological Signals pp. 339–356" published by Springer © 1996)

trode which could be a surface type located at a remote site of the body, the recording area from this electrode is circular and potentials are larger and longer than other needle electrodes. Primarily because more muscle fibers are within the zone of detection. The bipolar electrode has two platinum wires and a grounded outer shaft. The recording range of the bipolar electrode is restricted to the area between two wires. Therefore, it is unsatisfactory for routine clinical practice. The concentric needle consists of an outer shaft serving as a local reference electrode, and an inner electrode wire embedded in the bevel of the needle. Because the electrode cannula acts as a shield, the electrode has directional recording characteristics depending on the angle and position of the needle bevel. The recorded potentials are smaller and shorter than those recorded with monopolar needle electrode. In the single fiber electrode, the reference is the cut end of a wire embedded in a hole in the side of the needle shaft, 3 mm from the tip. It is the most sensitive test to demonstrate an impaired neuromuscular transmission like myasthenia gravis but it needs considerable experience and technical expertise [10]. The hooked wire electrode needle contained two hooked wire electrodes inside an insertion needle. When the needle is withdrawn, the hook on the end of the wire acts as a barb, stabilizing the position in the muscle. It could be left in place for long periods of time such as hours or even days.

The author use monopolar needle electrode routinely for clinical practice after considering the aforementioned characteristics of different needles. There are also various injection needle electrodes that could be used for diagnosing and injection simultaneously such as (Bo-ject Disposable Needle Electrode, Alpine Biomed ApS, Skovlunde, Denmark) and (Ambu® Neuroline Inoject, Ambu A/S, Baltorpbakken 13, DK-2750 Ballerup)

12.2.3 Preparation and Insertion of Needle Electrode

The laryngeal EMG could be performed easily and safely. The author uses injection monopolar needle electrode as thin as 25 or 26 gauge that looks like an acupuncture needle. Although it is thin but is feasible for injecting augmentation materials such as hyaluronic acid. Because local anesthesia may alter laryngeal EMG results (especially in cricothyroid muscle), and the procedure is generally not very painful, local anesthesia is not used. The patient is placed in the supine position with a soft pillow under the shoulder and the neck extended. The posture of cervical extension facilitates localization of the puncture site at the cricothyroid (CT) notch. Before inserting the needle electrode, a surface electrode could be placed at neck closed to clavicle and it is used as the ground electrode. Another surface electrode could be placed on the cheek and it works as reference electrode. After cleaning the skin with alcohol, the CT notch just above cricoid cartilage could be localized by palpation. The needle is inserted through the skin approximately 0.5 cm from the midline. The aforementioned CT muscle and TA/LCA muscle could be punctured and tested to reflect the function of SLN and RLN respectively.

12.2.3.1 Cricothyroid (CT) Muscle

The cricothyroid (CT) muscle could be punctured by angling the needle laterally 45° with 1 cm deep aiming at the junction point of lower margin and oblique line of thyroid cartilage (Fig. 12.3). To validate the position of the electrode in CT muscle, the patient is asked to phonate vowel/i/at a low pitch and then a high pitch. If the electrode is right in place, the EMG activity increases sharply. The diagnostic information therefore could be collected to represent the function of superior laryngeal nerve according to later description.

12.2.3.2 Thyroarytenoid and Lateral Cricoarytenoid (TA/LCA) Muscle Complex

To evaluate the thyroarytenoid (TA) and lateral cricoarytenoid (LCA) muscle complex, after puncturing CT muscle, the electrode needle tip is withdrawn slightly and the direction changed to superiorly and laterally 30° with 1–2 cm beneath the skin. The TA/LCA muscle complex is underneath the thyroid cartilage (Fig. 12.4). According to the dissection study of the level of anterior

Fig. 12.3 The cricothyroid (CT) muscle could be punctured by angling the needle laterally 45° via cricothyroid membrane and EMG obtained from CT muscle reflect the function of superior laryngeal nerve

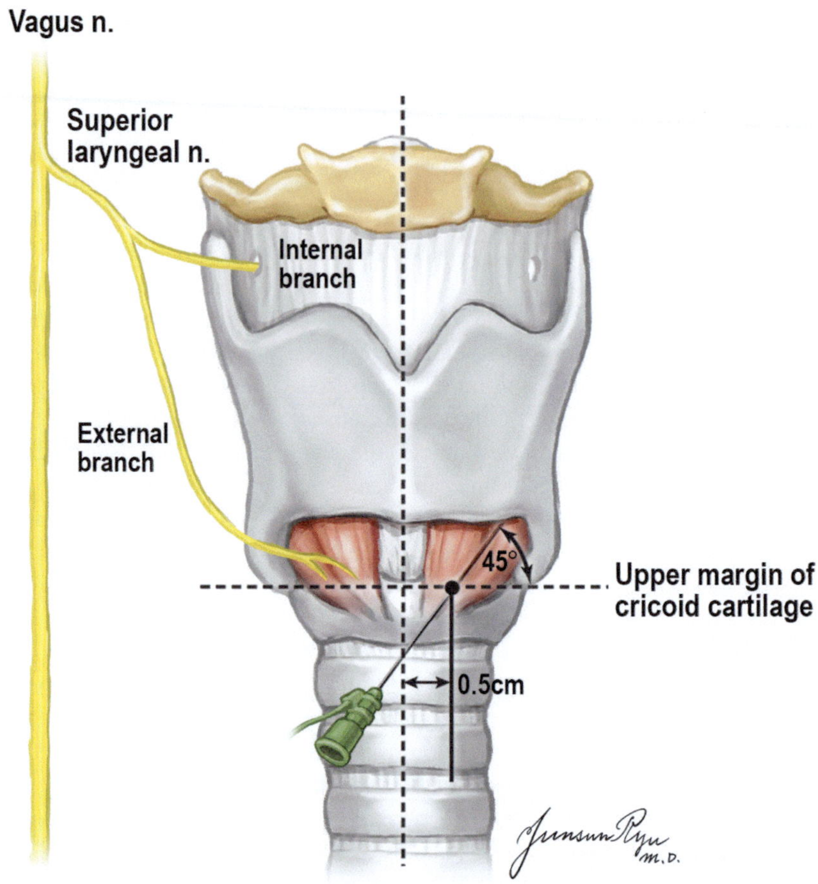

commissure of the larynx, [11] the mean distance of vocal fold from the lower margin of thyroid cartilage was 10.54 ± 1.73 mm in male and 9.38 ± 3.43 mm in female. The length of membranous vocal fold was 15.00 ± 3.18 mm in male and 12.88 ± 4.12 mm in female. Another anatomical study evaluated 2 CT membrane approaches by using cadaver larynx with skin and soft tissue removed. The needle was inserted into vocal fold muscle just inferior to the lower margin of thyroid cartilage by infrathyroid approach or just superior to the upper margin of cricoids cartilage by supracricoid approach. The mean insertion depth from CT membrane was 11.3 ± 1.8 mm for infrathyroid approach, which was significantly less than the depth for the supracricoid approach (18.2 ± 2.4 mm) [12]. The aforementioned anatomical characters could be used as a reference to help puncture the TA/LCA complex.

The author puts the finger along the lower margin of thyroid cartilage during the procedure and feels the needle goes just underneath the thyroid cartilage. If the needle is too superficial, surgeon's finger may feel the motion of the needle. When the needle was located outside the thyroid cartilage and in the strap muscle, muscle action potential will be induced if patient was asked to up and down chin. The signal induced by aforementioned motion confirms the mis-placement of the needle. Contrarily, triggering of a cough during inserting a needle generally indicates that the needle has penetrated the airway and is causing irritation of the mucosa. In such case of too deep insertion, the needle should be withdrawn. While the tip of the needle is in right place of TA/LCA complex, the position of the needle is validated by asking the patient to say and sustain the vowel/i/with increase in EMG activity.

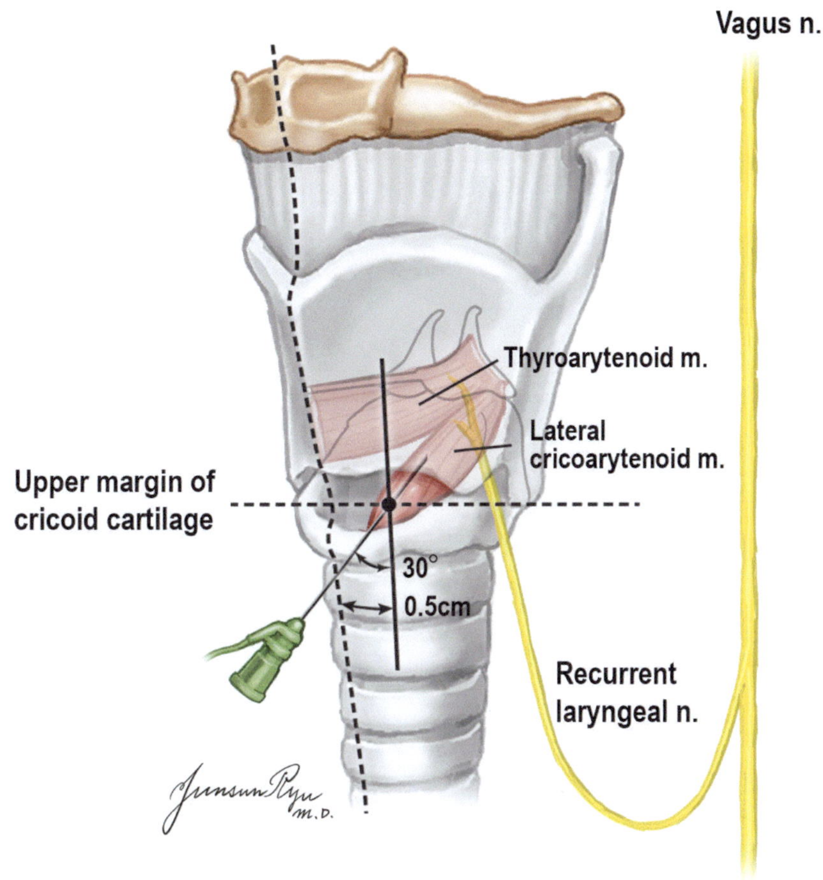

Fig. 12.4 The thyroarytenoid/lateral cricoarytenoid (TA/LCA) muscle complex could be punctured by angling the needle laterally 30° via cricothyroid membrane and EMG obtained from TA/LCA muscle reflect the function of recurrent laryngeal nerve

12.2.4 Basic Interpretation of EMG

We can interpret the EMG by observing the appearance of muscle activity on monitor and listen to the sound of the activity transmitted through a speaker. The frequencies of muscle action potentials range between 2 and 10,000 Hz and the frequency band of the EMG machine is typically set at 10–10,000 Hz.

Because the needle itself has some electrical energy, a burst of electrical signal is produced while the needle is inserted into the muscle. The signal is insertional activity and should last no more than several hundred milliseconds [8]. However, there is no literature reporting using the insertional activity to predict prognosis of UVFP. According to the experience of author, the signal is too short to be well recorded. Therefore, laryngeal EMG is performed and evaluated mainly in two parts: (1) the muscle at rest (ask the examined patient to keep silent) and (2) during muscle voluntary contraction (ask the examined patient to phonate vowel/i/.

12.2.4.1 In the Muscle at Rest (Keep Silent)

Theoretically, normal resting muscle is silent but patients often have difficulty completely relaxing a muscle. The motor unit activity associated with incomplete relaxation is distinguished from abnormal spontaneous activity by its rhythmicity. Spontaneous activity refers to the presence of electrical activity in severely denervated, unstable resting muscles. The presence of spontaneous activity implies that the muscle is degenerating or that the nerve has been injured and the process that caused the injury is ongoing. Because of the length of time it takes for enough degeneration to

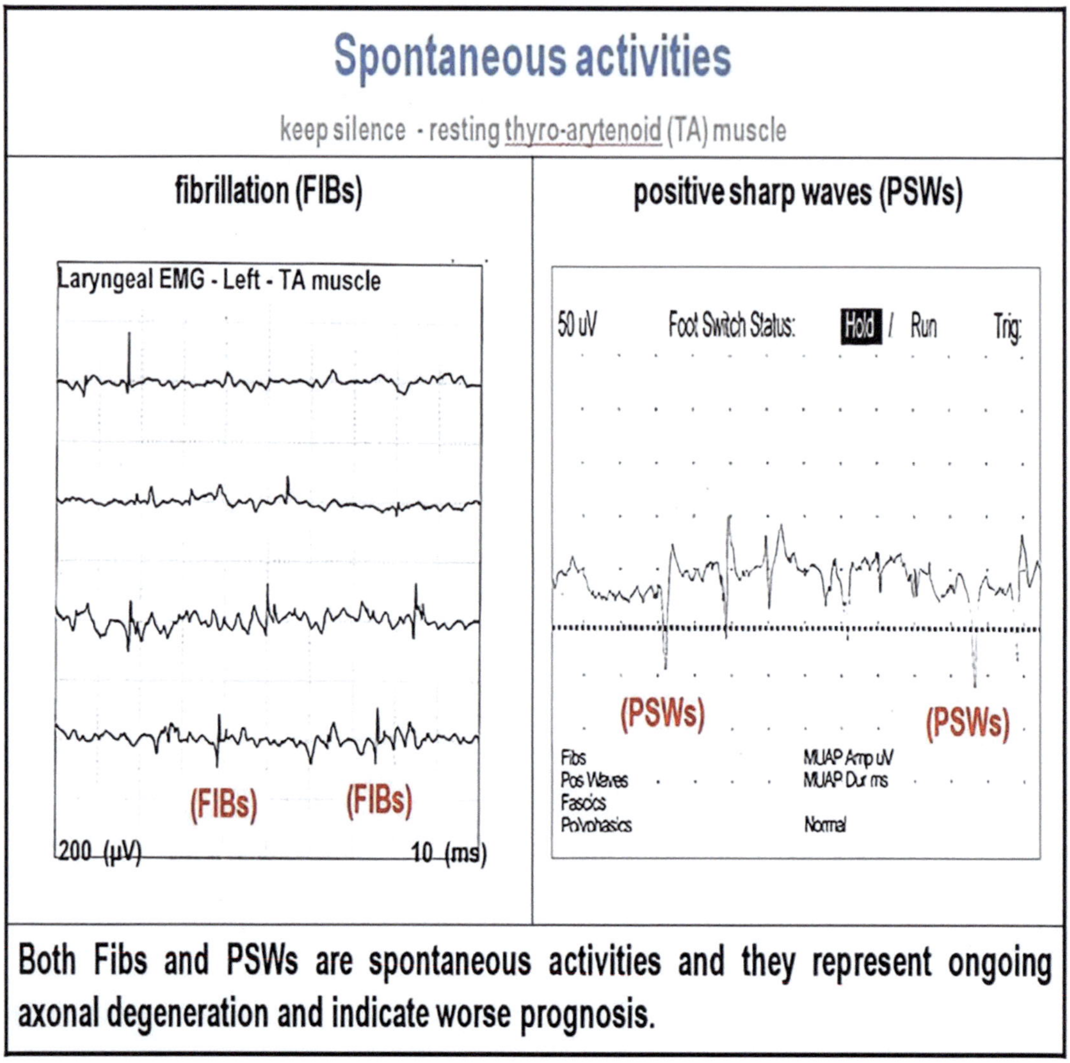

Fig. 12.5 Fibrillation potentials (FIBs) and positive sharp waves (PSWs) are spontaneous activities and they represent ongoing axonal degeneration and indicate worse prognosis

occur to cause an absence of electrical impulses from the nerve to the muscle, spontaneous activity usually begins 2–3 weeks after denervation has occurred [8]. Therefore, LEMG is recommended at least 2 weeks after onset of symptoms of unilateral vocal fold paralysis.

According to the experience of author, the most common spontaneous activity during testing paralyzed vocal fold is fibrillation potentials (fibs), which are the action potentials of single muscle fibers that are firing spontaneously in the absence of innervations. Typically they have a regular firing pattern at rates of 1–50 Hz, with amplitude of several hundred microvolts and duration of less than 2 ms (Fig. 12.5). The amplitude is variable and is proportional to the fiber diameter. The fibs have a characteristic rhythmic sound transmitted through a loud speaker. The typical sound allows one to identify the fibs even without looking at the oscilloscope screen of EMG machine. Because fibs sounds like "machine gun firing" or "rain drop on the roof.". The typical sound is easy to remember and very helpful to identify the fibs during laryngeal EMG.

There are several other spontaneous activities such as positive sharp wave, complex repetitive discharge, myotonic potentials, fasciculation potentials, myokymic discharges, neuromyotonic discharges, cramp potentials. Positive sharp waves and fibs usually occur together. The other spontaneous activities are rarely seen in EMG for vocal fold paralysis. Readers could refer to the paper of Yolanda et al. [8] and Mills [13], the textbook edited by Sataloff et al. [9] or the internet [14] for details of aforementioned signals.

12.2.4.2 In the Muscle at Voluntary Contraction (Phonating Vowel/I/)

By asking patient to phonate with lower pitch (CT muscle) or lower intensity (TA-LCA complex), the intrinsic laryngeal muscles contract minimally and allow us to observe the waveform morphology of recruited motor unit potentials (MUPs). A number of parameters of MUPs could be measured such as amplitude, duration, number of phases (changes in direction), and firing rate etc [13]. The normal MUPs of laryngeal muscles are usually biphasic or triphasic with an initial downward positive spike. The normal MUPs have amplitude ranged from 200 to 500 microvolts and duration of 5–6 ms [8]. The amplitude of the MUPs reflects the number and the strength of the muscle fibers innervated by one nerve ending. The duration of the MUPs reflects the velocity of the neural input, which is influenced by insulation of the nerves. After injury, the nerve undergoes a process of denervation followed by regeneration. During the early phases of regeneration, the combination of minimally insulated nerves and weak muscle fibers produces MUPs that have small amplitude, long duration, and polyphasic shapes on laryngeal EMG. As the regeneration progresses, not all of the neurons regenerate, those neurons that regenerate therefore branch more than before the injury to innervate as many muscle fibers that lack innervation as possible. The MUPs are usually described as giant polyphasic MUPs with polyphasic morphology, greater amplitude, and prolonged duration. The presence of this signal implies and old nerve injury [8].

When the patient was asked to phonate with increased pitch or intensity, more motor units are recruited and potentials overlap and interfere with each other; hence this is sometimes referred to as the interference pattern. But recruitment pattern is now the preferred term [13]. Recruitment reflects the degree of innervations and effective recruitment is seen on laryngeal EMG as an increase in the number and density of motor unit potentials. We could compare the recruitment pattern of the paralyzed vocal fold to the normal mobile vocal fold and estimate the percentage of recruitment reduction (RR) (Fig. 12.6).

12.2.5 Laryngeal EMG and Prognosis of Unilateral Vocal Fold Paralysis

The decision-making algorithm for the management of patients with UVFP has always been complex. In this algorithm, severity of symptoms, the vocal needs of the patient, and prognostic data are usually most important. Accurate prognostic information is important for the physician to determine the type and timing of surgical intervention to be used. In literature, several studies used laryngeal EMG to predict the prognosis with different methodologies and results [15–19]. The meta-analysis of Rickert et al. [20] concluded that laryngeal EMG is not useful in predicting recovery from UVFP, as it is compromised by the characteristic and complex aspects of laryngeal reinnervation such as synkinesis. But it is an accurate and useful tool for predicting failure of recovery in those who presents laryngeal EMG signals of severe nerve injury.

According to literature, the aforementioned spontaneous activities and reduced recruitment pattern recorded by laryngeal EMG was most commonly used as poor prognostic factors for patients of UVFP. The author had published a long-term prospective study with level 1b evidence in year 2015 [19]. In our definition, in comparing the normal side laryngeal EMG, if the paralyzed vocal fold TA/LCA muscle complex had >20% recruitment reduction (RR) during task of phonation and/or spontaneous activity during task of keeping silent, the laryngeal EMG result is positive and the prognosis of vocal fold motion recovery is poor. The positive predictive value is as high as 97.9% especially when the laryngeal EMG was done at more than 2 months

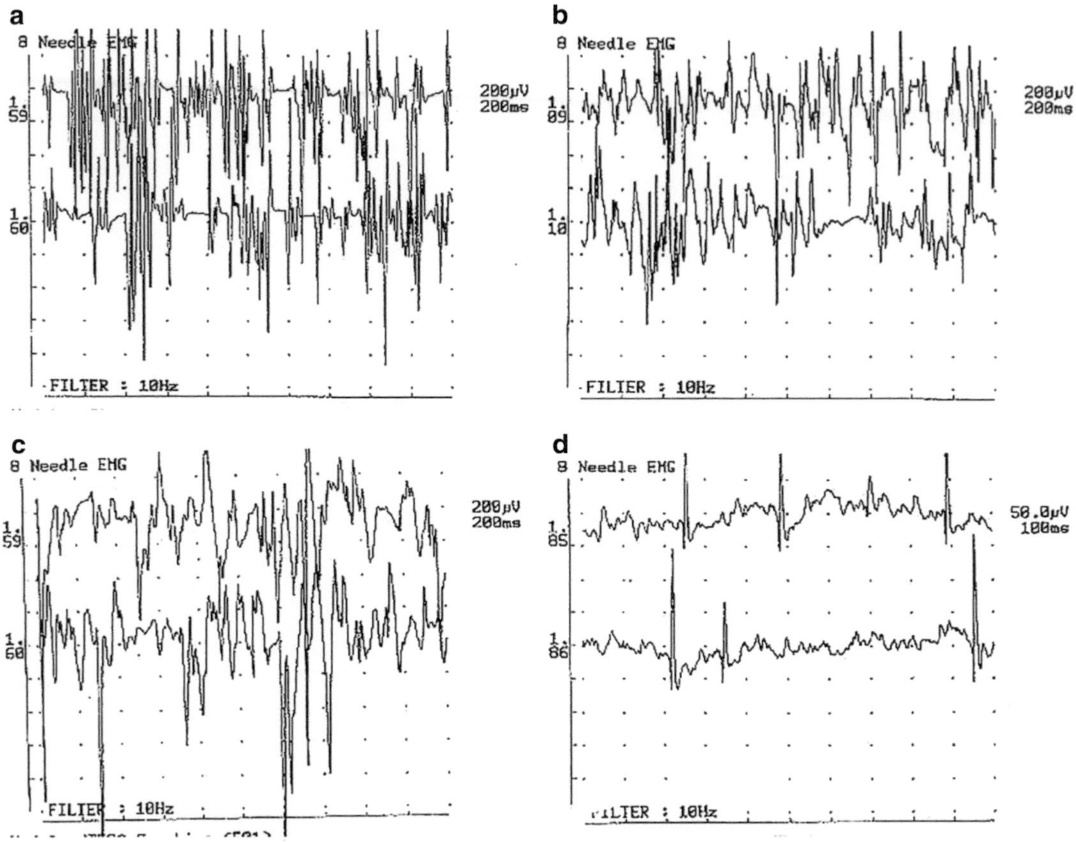

Fig. 12.6 The recruitment pattern of TA/LCA muscle complex in normal and paralyzed vocal folds. (**a**) full recruitment in normal vocal fold (**b**) about 30% recruitment reduction in paralyzed vocal fold (**c**) about 50% recruitment reduction in paralyzed vocal fold (**d**) about 90% recruitment reduction in paralyzed vocal fold

after symptoms onset of UVFP. Permanent laryngeal framework surgery may be executed as early as possible if the results of conservative speech therapy or minimal invasive injection laryngoplasty is not satisfactory.

12.3 Laryngeal EMG Guided Injection Laryngoplasty for UVFP

One of the mainstay of surgical treatment of UVFP is displacing the paralyzed vocal fold toward the midline of glottis to facilitate glottal closure. In addition to medialization laryngoplasty, injection laryngoplasty or vocal fold injection discussed in this textbook is a popular minimal invasive treatment since it was developed by Bruening in 1911 [21]. Traditionally, vocal fold injection was performed under the guidance of direct or indirect laryngoscopy. According to the review of Sulica et al. in 2010, [22] awake vocal fold injection under flexible laryngoscope guidance and the transcricothyroid membrane approach (47%) is the most often used technique in USA nowadays. However, this technique needs a perfect cooperation between the injected patient, surgeon and assistant handling the scope. Sometimes, the injection is not easy and developing another method of guidance in office-based service is necessary.

12.3.1 Rationale of Laryngeal EMG Guided Injection Laryngoplasty

In 1988, Ludlow et al. started using laryngeal EMG to administer botulinum toxin injection into the TA muscle to treat adductor spasmodic dysphonia and laryngeal EMG has been widely used in guiding this treatment modality although there is no specific laryngeal EMG signal for adductor spasmodic dysphonia. Because the TA muscle is also the vocal fold injection target for UVFP, it is reasonable that laryngeal EMG could be used to guide some commercially available forgiving injectable substance like hyaluronic acid in vocal fold injection.

Skepticism about laryngeal EMG guided injection laryngoplasty mainly comes from loss of visual monitoring in the approach. However, patient discomfort accounted for the largest group of injection failure in awake subjects according to the review of Sulica et al. [22] Patient anxiety and a strong gag reflex that persists through topical anesthesia are general contraindications for flexible laryngoscopy guided injection. Thorough nasal and larynx local anesthesia is important but Sulica et al. have noted that it is possible to anesthetize excessively, causing salivary secretions to overwhelm the larynx, making the patient uncomfortable and obscuring the injection site. In addition, the view of atrophic paralyzed vocal fold could also be blocked by compensatory hypertrophic false vocal fold in some patients (Fig. 12.7). In the aforementioned most popular transcricothyroid membrane needle approach, the transcervical submucosa passage of the needle still cannot be seen directly even with video-chip laryngoscopy. Sulica et al. reminded us that the location of the needle depends on identification of transmitted motion within the vocal fold by laryngoscopy, which sometimes proves difficult. Therefore, visual guidance is not always optimal and electrical signal guidance could be an alternative. Similar to bats hunt in the dark using echolocation, we may use the aforementioned electrical signal to localize the paralyzed TA/LCA muscle complex and deliver augmentation materials into it. The author has published the technique in year 2012 [23] (Fig. 12.8).

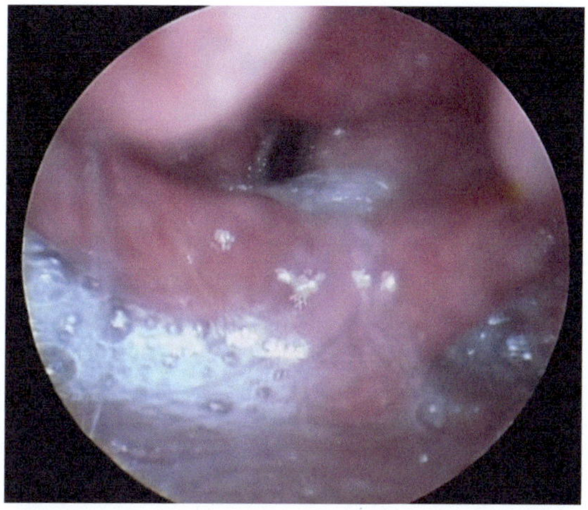

Fig. 12.7 During flexible laryngoscopy, saliva secretion overwhelming the larynx, supraglottic contraction, or strong gagp reflex is not uncommon in patients of unilateral vocal fold paralysis and vocal fold injection augmentation may be difficult under laryngoscopy guidance

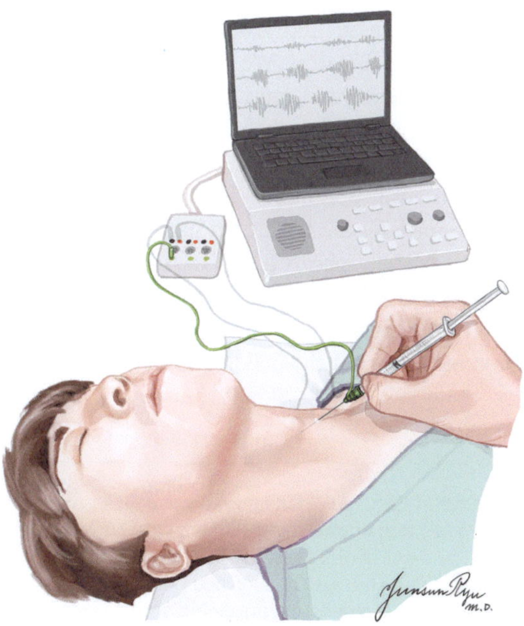

Fig. 12.8 Vocal fold injection augmentation via an injectable needle electrode during laryngeal EMG without the need of flexible laryngoscopy guidance. The technique combines prognosis evaluation and treatment of unilateral vocal fold paralysis in one step. (Figure was redrawn based on [32] with permission)

12.3.2 Procedure of Laryngeal EMG Guided Injection Laryngoplasty

The procedure of the injection is similar to the steps aforementioned in performing laryngeal EMG. There is a “rule of two” for readers to remember the procedure easily. Simply speaking, we puncture the larynx at “2” sides starting from normal vocal fold and then paralyzed vocal fold.

In each side, we puncture "2" muscles starting from CT muscle and then TA/LCA muscle complex. In each muscle we ask patient to do "2" tasks including keeping silent and phonation to collect possible existed "2" signals such as spontaneous activities or recruitment reduction. When the needle tip is finally inserted into the paralyzed TA/LCA muscle, we carefully listen to the speaker to detect any fibrillation potentials which is the best signal to ensure the needle is in the paralyzed muscle. We then ask the patient to phonate and record the recruitment pattern. A significant recruitment reduction also confirms the needle is in paralyzed muscle. Surgeon's left hand fix the needle in place to avoid movement, a 1-ml syringe of hyaluronic acid (HA) was connected to the injectable needle electrode. The patient was asked to keep silent, avoid swallowing saliva. Surgeon's right hand pushes 0.5 ml of HA into the muscle complex. We ask the patient to phonate again and listen to the voice that becomes less breathy. We ensure the needle is still in the paralyzed muscle by aforementioned two tasks and inject the last 0.5 ml of HA (Fig. 12.9).

Fibrillation potentials (fibs) and recruitment reduction (RR) are both obvious signals to help localize the paralyzed TA/LCA muscle. However, if there were no fibs and recruitment pattern during phonation is nearly normal, surgeon may suspect the needle is misplaced in the normal contracted strap muscle. The patient could be asked to up and down his/her chin; this maneuver should activate MUPs if the needle is misplaced in strap muscle. Otherwise, the needle is in TA/LCA muscle and laryngeal EMG with nearly normal recruitment indicates good prognosis. In rare cases of a patient with electrical silence and no recruitment during patient's phonation, the signal also confirms the needle in right place and indicate poor prognosis. In our experience, when we falsely punctured the needle tip into the airway during patient's phonation of vowel/i/, the speaker broadcasted the patient's voice louder and it sounded like the patient was using a microphone. In addition, irritation of airway mucosa will induce patient's cough and needle should be withdrawn to relocate to a right place.

12.3.3 Injection Material, Volume, and Effect Duration

There is several injection materials could be used and discussion is done in Chap. 10. Briefly speaking, Ideal VFI material should be biocompatible, biomechanically similar to vocal fold components, easily injectable through a fine needle, readily available with minimal preparation time, applicable in an outpatient setting, resistant to absorption or migration, and easily removable in

Fig. 12.9 LEMG guided hyaluronic acid (HA) vocal fold injection for a patient with left vocal fold paralysis
(**a**) Open phase of glottis, the fixed left arytenoid is marked by x
(**b**) Closed phase of glottis, the fixed left arytenoid is marked by x and there was a large glottal gap between 2 vocal folds while the patient phonated
(**c**) A 26-gauge monopolar injectable needle electrode was inserted through cricothyroid membrane into the TA/LCA muscle of normal right side vocal fold
(**d**) The LEMG on the unaffected right side vocal fold showed a normal motor unit potential recruitment pattern
(**e**) The needle electrode was withdrawn and then inserted through the cricothyroid membrane again into the paralyzed left side TA/LCA muscle. While the patient was silent, fibrillations signal could be seen (arrows). While the patient phonated, reduced recruitment was noticed (not shown in the image)
(**f**) Before completion of LEMG, 1.0cc of HA was injected via the injectable needle electrode into the paralyzed TA/LCA muscle
(**g**) Open phase of glottis after the injection, the fixed left arytenoid is marked by x and left vocal fold was augmented with HA (arrow)
(**h**) Closed phase of glottis after the injection, the fixed left arytenoid is marked by x. The glottis could be closed well after the injection

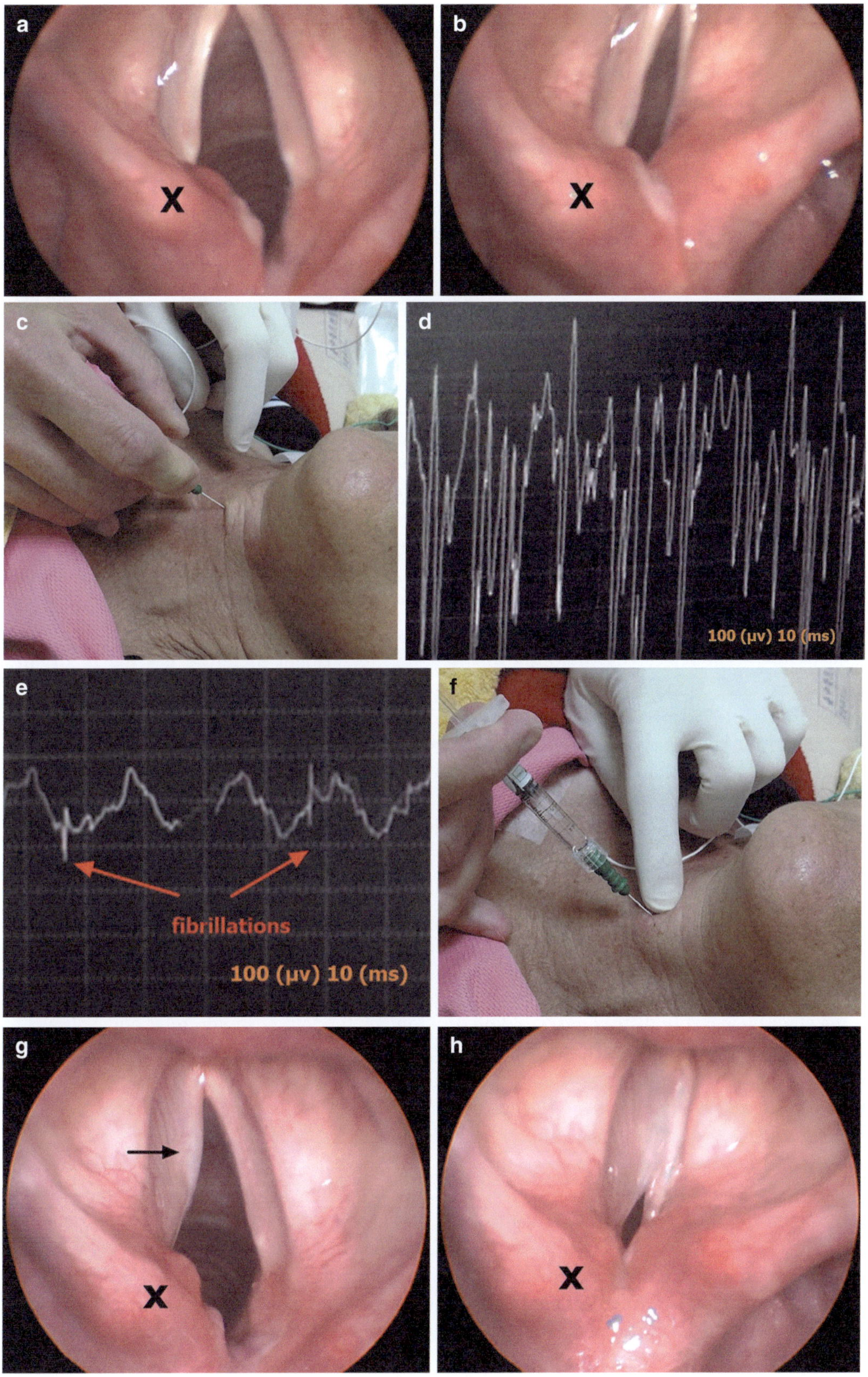
a
X
b
X
c
d
100 (μv) 10 (ms)
e
fibrillations
100 (μv) 10 (ms)
f
g
X
h
X

the event of revision surgery [24]. Hyaluronic acid (HA) is an augmentation material that fulfills all of the aforementioned requirements except the problem of absorption and the author uses it in clinical practice.

Two commercially available HA are commonly used. Hylaform is created from rooster combs. Restylane is a non-animal, stabilized hyaluronic acid (NASHA), which is biotechnologically generated by Streptococcus species of bacteria. Both were developed as dermal filler, but the study of Caton [25] showed Hylaform and Restylane share comparable elastic values and low viscosity that are similar to cadaveric vocal fold. They both have family products of different particles sizes. For example, Hylaform had smaller particle size similar to Restylane. Hylaform plus and Restylane Perlane are cross-linked HA that has larger particle sizes. Results from the study by Lau [26] show that large particle size HA is more durable than small particle HA for IL. The author of this chapter Wang et al. also reported using Restylane Perlane and obtained long-term effect (mean follow up of 16.2 months) after one injection in most of their patients [27]. Gotxi-Erezuma et al. also reported HA injection laryngoplasty by EMG and their patients had significant improvement after 6 months follow up in their study [28].

Readers might be concerned about the adequate injected volume of HA needed to obtain a satisfactory result. According to literature, the mean injected volume is usually less than 1 ml [23] and 1 ml injection was usually enough to achieve overcorrection of a paralyzed vocal fold. Sulica et al. [22] described that "In the event that the injectant is unevenly distributed, yielding an irregular or lump vocal fold contour, a throat clear, or a sharp cough by the patient usually helps to distribute it more evenly." Because the shape of the overinjected vocal fold will be remodeled in response to the compression from the contralateral mobile vocal fold, delicate visual monitoring of the vocal fold HA injection amount and injection site by laryngoscopy will become less important. The author routinely injected 1 ml of HA, if 1 ml HA failed to close the very large glottal gap in some patients, laryngeal framework surgery will be considered if EMG indicated poor prognosis.

There are three main rationales for an absorbable hyaluronic acid injection to have a long-term augmentation effect in our practice. First, Restylane Perlane undergoes isovolemic degradation by which it aggregates more water as it is absorbed; hence, it can maintain the volume in the injection area for a longer period than an autologous transplant [29]. In addition, an animal study showed that injected VF was stimulated by HA to regenerate collagen and endogenous HA that replaces the absorbed HA volume [30]. Second, there is a strong propensity for laryngeal reinnervation after VFP. Preferential reinnervation of paralyzed adductor muscles may account for a medial position of the paralyzed VF. The atrophic thyroarytenoid muscle could also regain some muscle bulk after the regeneration [31]. Third, during the gradual absorption of injected HA in some of our patients, the contralateral healthy VF probably compensated for the glottis closure. From the aforementioned reasons, the injected patient therefore has the possibility to have long-term recovery of voice after one minimal injection shot.

12.3.4 Algorithm of EMG Guided Injection Laryngoplasty for UVFP

As mentioned previously, European Laryngological Society commented that many laryngologists do not routinely use laryngeal EMG because of a persistent lack of agreement on methodology, interpretation, validity, and clinical application of this technique [7]. To enhance the clinical popularity of laryngeal EMG, the author proposed aforementioned EMG guided injection laryngoplasty for UVFP as an innovative implementation of laryngeal EMG [32]. By this way, evaluation, prognosis prediction and treatment for UVFP could be achieved in one step and the technique could be adopted as a routine initial management of UVFP. The algorithm of the technique is shown in Fig. 12.10. In brief, if patient had short-term injection augmen-

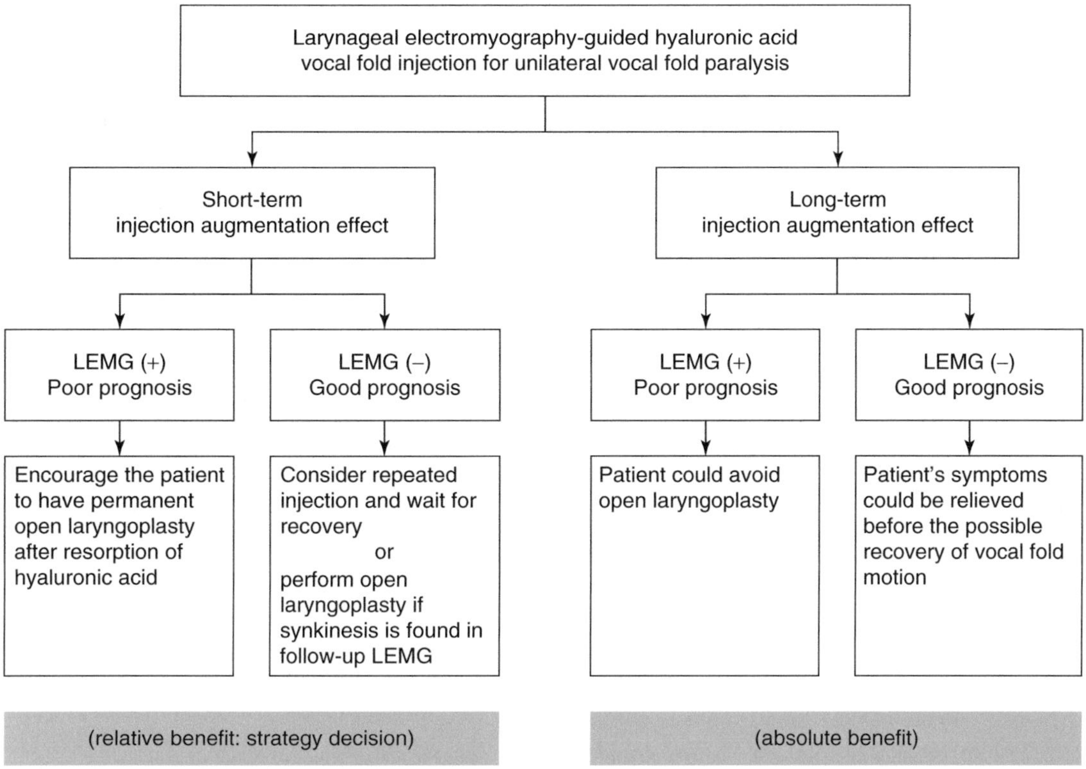

Fig. 12.10 The algorithm of laryngeal EMG guided hyaluronic acid vocal fold injection for unilateral vocal fold paralysis. (Figure was used with permission from [32])

tation effect, the data of laryngeal EMG could be used to predict prognosis and for consultation of future management. Contrarily, if patient obtained long-term effect, they will be happy about sparing the possible open laryngeal framework surgery and the routinely collected data could be used for research and therefore improving our understanding of this disease entity. The benefits for both doctors and patients should enhance the value and popularity of laryngeal EMG. From the merit of this innovative management, the author has done several researches based on this strategy [19, 23, 27, 33–35].

12.4 Consultation Cautions and Limitations

Although the feasibility of EMG guided injection laryngoplasty has been approved by our study, there is still no standard procedure for vocal fold injection so far and different vocal fold injection methods have different pros and cons. Similar to other techniques, there are several cautions and limitations of EMG guided injection laryngoplasty that surgeons need to know to give patients best consultation.

The first and most important caution is the injected patient of UVFP needs to be confirmed to have a fully abducted vocal fold during inspiration on the healthy side by laryngeal videostroboscopy. Therefore the 1 ml injection augmentation shall not cause airway problem even without visual monitoring. This principle is approved by the author's injection for more than 300 patients without airway problem. To avoid hematoma formation on patients with bleeding tendency, anticoagulant medication is recommended to be discontinued at least 1 week before injection. If the patient's cricothyroid membrane could not be well identified by palpation at consultation, EMG guided injection laryngoplasty is also contraindicated. For example, patients with obese neck, severe lymph edema caused by irradiation, hypertrophic scar, etc. are not good candidates to receive this treatment.

Before injection, possible absorption of HA and loss of augmentation effect in the future should be mentioned to the patients although there is also chance for them to get long-term effect. After injection, if the augmentation effect in some patients is not permanent, the trial augmentation is not harmful for those patients because they will understand the expected benefits of open laryngeal framework surgery and the laryngeal EMG data will be used to help them to make a decision for further salvage treatment. After injection, there is no need for patients to do voice rest. Theoretically, the HA is deeply injected to the TA/LCA muscle and the vibrating cover layer of vocal fold is not influenced by the injection. In fact, normal speech is encouraged promptly after injection and the shape of the injected vocal fold shall be remodeled in response to the compression from the contralateral mobile vocal fold. Speech therapy could be done immediately after injection to help patients to phonate efficiently. Because the injection needle is 26 Gauge thin and pain is usually minimal, pain killer is optional. In the practice of author, patients were followed up at 1 month, 3 months, and 6 months after injection. After a half year follow-up, the patient could be followed every 6 months or they could come back promptly once symptoms recurred.

In conclusion, otolaryngologists continue to use a variety of techniques to perform vocal fold injection. The choice of technique is usually based on surgeon preference. Each surgeon tended to adopt one particular method after initial trials of several other techniques. The aforementioned EMG guided injection laryngoplasty has several advantages and is the only management that could provide patient prognostic information simultaneously with injection augmentation. The author recommends this technique as an early initial minimal invasive management for patient with UVFP. For surgeons who used to do endoscopic guided injection, EMG guided injection could also be reserved to salvage failure in patients with visual monitoring difficulty.

Key Learning Points:

- Laryngeal electromyography (EMG) is the only test that can provide laryngologists with the neuromuscular status and prognostic information of patients with unilateral vocal fold paralysis (UVFP).
- We could follow the "rule of two" for performing laryngeal EMG.
  - Two disciplines: laryngologists cooperate with neurologists.
  - Two sides checkup: normal side and paralyzed side larynx.
  - Two muscles be punctured: cricothyroid (CT) muscle reflect the function of superior laryngeal nerve; thyroarytenoid/lateral cricoarytenoid (TA/LCA) muscle complex reflect the function of recurrent laryngeal nerve.
  - Two tasks: ask the patient to keep silent and ask the patient to phonate vowel/i/.
  - Two signals: the fibrillation signals when patient is silent and the recruitment pattern when patient phonates could be used for predicting the prognosis of UVFP.
- In comparing the normal side laryngeal EMG, if the paralyzed vocal fold TA/LCA muscle complex had >20% recruitment reduction (RR) during task of phonation and/or spontaneous activity during task of keeping silent, the laryngeal EMG result is positive and the prognosis of vocal fold motion recovery is poor.
- Before finishing the laryngeal EMG, 1 ml of hyaluronic acid could be delivered through a thin monopolar injectable needle electrode into the TA/LCA muscle complex of paralyzed vocal fold via the transcervical cricothyroid membrane puncture under laryngeal EMG guidance. The injection augmentation for UVFP could be performed simultaneously with laryngeal EMG.
- Before this practice, full abduction of healthy side vocal fold during inspira-

tion should be confirmed by laryngeal videostroboscopy.

- For patients who could not obtain long-term augmentation effect after injection, the laryngeal EMG information could be used for guiding future management. For example, thyroplasty type I could be performed early if prognosis is poor.
- This laryngeal EMG guided injection laryngoplasty is a feasible initial management for UVFP. Diagnosis, treatment and prognosis prediction could be finished in one shot.

References

1. Yamada M, Hirano M, Ohkubo H. Recurrent laryngeal nerve paralysis: a 10-year review of 564 patients. Auris Nasus Larynx. 1983;10(Suppl):S1–S15.
2. Havas T, Lowinger D, Priestley J. Unilateral vocal fold paralysis: causes, options and outcomes. Aust N Z J Surg. 1999;69:509–13.
3. Siu J, Tam S, Fung KA. Comparison of outcomes in interventions for unilateral vocal fold paralysis: a systematic review. Laryngoscope. 2016;126(7):1616–24.
4. Weddel GB, Pattle RE. The electrical activity of voluntary muscle in man under normal and pathological conditions. Brain. 1944;67:178–257.
5. Faaborg-Andersen K. Action potentials from internal laryngeal muscles during phonation. Nature. 1956;177(4503):340–1.
6. Buchthal F. Electromyography of intrinsic laryngeal muscles. Q J Exp Physiol Cogn Med Sci. 1959;44(2):137–48.
7. Volk GF, Hagen R, Pototschnig C, et al. Laryngeal electromyography: a proposal for guidelines of the European laryngological society. Eur Arch Otorhinolaryngol. 2012;269:2227–45.
8. Yolanda D, Heman-Ackah YD, Mandel S, Manon-Espaillat R, Abaza MM, Sataloff RT. Laryngeal electromyography. Otolaryngol Clin North Am. 2007;40(5):1003–23., vi-vii. https://doi.org/10.1016/j.otc.2007.05.007.
9. Sataloff RT, Mandel S, Heman-Ackah Y, et al. Laryngeal electromyography. 2nd ed. San Diego: Plural Publishing, Inc.; 2006. p. 54.
10. Selvan VA. Single-fiber EMG: a review. Ann Indian Acad Neurol. 2011;14(1):64–7.
11. Ortug G, Liman Z, Ortug A. A Dissectional study of the level of anterior commissure of the larynx. Ear Nose Throat J. 2020;10:145561320931213. https://doi.org/10.1177/0145561320931213.
12. Panossian H, Pasick LJ, Sataloff RT. Anatomical study of two cricothyroid approaches to the cadaver larynx. J Voice. 2019:S0892–1997(19)30439–4.
13. Mills KR. The basics of electromyography. J Neurol Neurosurg Psychiatry. 2005;76(Suppl 2):32–5.
14. Abnormal spontaneous electromyographic activity. Long Davalos; Hani Kushlaf. NCBI StatPearls [Internet]. https://www.ncbi.nlm.nih.gov/books/NBK482461/
15. Hirano M, Nosoe I, Shin T, Maeyama T. Electromyography for laryngeal paralysis. In: Hirano M, Kirchner J, Bless D, editors. Neurolaryngology: recent advances. 1st ed. Boston, MA: College Hill; 1987. p. 232–48.
16. Sittel C, Stennert E, Thumfart WF, Dapunt U, Eckel HE. Prognostic value of laryngeal electromyography in vocal fold paralysis. Arch Otolaryngol Head Neck Surg. 2001;127(2):155–60.
17. Munin MC, Rosen CA, Zullo T. Utility of laryngeal electromyography in predicting recovery after vocal fold paralysis. Arch Phys Med Rehabil. 2003;84(8):1150–3.
18. Wang CC, Chang MH, Wang CP, Liu SA. Prognostic indicators of unilateral vocal fold paralysis. Arch Otolaryngol Head Neck Surg. 2008;134:380–8.
19. Wang CC, Chang MH, De Virgilio A, Jiang RS, Lai HC, Wang CP, Wu SH, Liu SA. Laryngeal electromyography and prognosis of unilateral vocal fold paralysis—a long-term prospective study. Laryngoscope. 2015;125(4):898–903. https://doi.org/10.1002/lary.24980.
20. Rickert SM, Childs LF, Carey BT, Murry T, Sulica L. Laryngeal electromyography for prognosis of vocal fold palsy: a meta-analysis. Laryngoscope. 2012;122(1):158–61.
21. Bruening W. Uber eine neue Behandlungs method der Rekurrenslahmung. Verh Dtsch Laryngol. 1911;18:23.
22. Sulica L, Rosen CA, Postma GN, Simpson B, Amin M, Courey M, Merati A. Current practice in injection augmentation of the vocal folds: indications, treatment principles, techniques, and complications. Laryngoscope. 2010;120:319–25.
23. Wang CC, Chang MH, Wang CP, Liu SA, Liang KL, Wu SH, Jiang RS, Huang HT, Lai HC. Laryngeal electromyography-guided hyaluronic acid vocal fold injection for unilateral vocal fold paralysis-preliminary results. J Voice. 2012;26(4):506–14.
24. Kwon TK, Buckmire R. Injection laryngoplasty for management of unilateral vocal fold paralysis. Curr Opin Otolaryngol Head Neck Surg. 2004;12:538–42.
25. Caton,T.; Thibeault, S.L.; Klemuk, S.; Smith, M.E. Viscoelasticity of hyaluronan and nonhyaluronan based vocal fold injectables: implications for mucosal versus muscle use Laryngoscope 2007; 117(3):516–521.
26. Lau DP, Lee GA, Wong SM, Lim VP, Chan YH, Tan NG, Rammage LA, Morrison MD. Injection Laryngoplasty with hyaluronic acid for unilateral vocal cord paralysis. Randomized controlled trial

comparing two different particle sizes. J Voice. 2010;24(1):113–8.
27. Wang CC, Chang MH, Jiang RS, Lai HC, De Virgilio A, Wang CP, Wu SH, Liu SA, Liang KL. Laryngeal electromyography-guided hyaluronic acid vocal fold injection for unilateral vocal fold paralysis- a prospective long term follow up outcome report. JAMA Otolaryngol Head Neck Surg. 2015;141(3):264–71.
28. Gotxi-Erezuma I, Ortega-Galán I, Laso-Elguezabal A, Puga, Bullido-Alonso C, García-Gutiérrez S, GP, Anton-Ladislao A, Moreno-Alonso E. Electromyography-guided hyaluronic acid injection Laryngoplasty in early stage of unilateral vocal fold paralysis. Acta Otorrinolaringol Esp 2017;68(5):274–283.
29. Friedman PM, Mafong EA, Kauvar AN, Geronemus RG. Safety data of injectable nonanimal stabilized hyaluronic acid gel for soft tissue augmentation. Dermatol Surg. 2002;28(6):491–4.
30. Hallen L, Johansson C, Laurent C. Cross-linked hyaluronan (Hylan B gel): a new injectable remedy for treatment of vocal fold insufficiency—an animal study. Acta Otolaryngol. 1999;119(1):107–11.
31. Woodson GE. Spontaneous laryngeal reinnervation after recurrent laryngeal or vagus nerve injury. Ann Otol Rhinol Laryngol. 2007;116(1):57–65.
32. Wang CC, Chang MH. A proposal to extend application of laryngeal electromyography (LEMG)-guided vocal fold injection to treatment of unilateral vocal fold paralysis to enhance clinical popularity of LEMG: response to the paper by G.F. Volk et al. Eur Arch Otorhinolaryngol. 2013;270:1563–5.
33. Hsieh YL, Chang MH, Wang CC. Laryngeal electromyography findings of vocal fold immobility in patients following radiotherapy for nasopharyngeal carcinoma. Head Neck. 2014;36(6):867–72.
34. De Virgilio A, Chang MH, Jiang RS, Wang CP, Wu SH, Liu SA, Wang CC. Influence of superior laryngeal nerve injury on glottal configuration/function of thyroidectomy-induced unilateral vocal fold paralysis. Otolaryngol Head Neck Surg. 2014;151(6):996–1002.
35. Wang CC. Reply to the effectiveness of using laryngeal EMG for injection augmentation. JAMA Otolaryngol Head Neck Surg. 2015;141(11):1030–1.

Ancillary Techniques for Vocal Fold Injection

13

Seong Keun Kwon

Abstract

Although conventional technique for vocal fold injection is widely used, several ancillary techniques have been reported to increase the accuracy of injection and be alternative in case of difficult laryngeal anatomy for conventional approach. While there has been limited literature report in terms of novel technique, a few techniques are used for clinical setting. In this chapter, author aims to introduce trans-nasal injection technique, light-guided injection technique, ultrasound-guided technique, and others.

Keywords

Trans-nasal approach · Ultrasound
Light-guided

13.1 Trans-Nasal Injection

A flexible endoscope with a working channel can be used for various laryngeal disease, such as evaluation of upper aerodigestive tract including the esophagus, biopsy for laryngeal and hypopharyngeal lesion, and laser ablation of laryngeal disease. Most of the procedure can be performed under local anesthesia. The preparation and setting of trans-nasal laryngeal injection are similar to other injection laryngoplasty technique; anesthesia to nose and pharynx [1]. Sufficient anesthesia of mucosa is the first step leading to the success of the procedure. The anesthesia of laryngeal mucosa can also be achieved by slow stalling of lidocaine above the vocal fold using fiberoptic injection needle through the working channel.

A flexible endoscope with a working channel usually has thicker diameter than those without working channel. For this reason, patients may complain the discomfort or pain on the nasal cavity and sufficient anesthesia and shrinkage of mucosa of nasal cavity should be performed before inserting the flexible endoscope (Table 13.1). In contrast, gag reflex and discomfort on the oropharynx may be less than trans-oral approach, because the injection needle does not pass through the oral cavity. Thus, trans-nasal laryngeal injection can be advantageous in those patients with strong gag reflex. Injection needle passes through the working channel and moves within the endoscopic view. The main operator manipulating the injection gauge and the assistant holding the endoscope should be cooperative for successful injection in trans-nasal approach. However, it is sometimes challenging when the main operator wants to separate the endoscopic view and approaching angle of the needle.

S. K. Kwon (✉)
Department of Otolaryngology Head and Neck Surgery, Seoul National University College of Medicine, Seoul, South Korea
e-mail: ent02@snu.ac.kr

© Springer Nature Singapore Pte Ltd. 2021

B.-J. Lee et al. (eds.), *Vocal Fold Injection*, https://doi.org/10.1007/978-981-16-3303-4_13

Table 13.1 The comparison of trans-oral and trans-nasal approaches

	Trans-oral approach	Trans-nasal approach
Discomfort on the oral cavity	+	–
Possible gag reflex[a]	+++	+
Discomfort on the nasal cavity	+	++
Approaching angle of needle	Can be separated from endoscopic view	Always moves with endoscopic view
Cooperation of main operator and endoscope holding assistant	+	+++

[a]Gag reflex can be minimized with sufficient anesthesia in both approaches

Several studies reported the feasibility of trans-nasal approach in injection laryngoplasty for unilateral vocal fold paralysis. Although the patients included in those studies are not numerous, the experiences with trans-nasal injection of various injection material, including fat and steroid, showed that this technique is a safe and efficacious phonosurgical procedure [2–5].

13.2 Light-Guided Injection

This technique is basically for transcutaneous approach, such as trans-thyrohyoid membrane, during which the tip of injection needle cannot be visualized. It has been postulated that it is necessary to develop expertise in correlating external landmarks with internal laryngeal anatomy for these blind approaches. In addition, a certain learning curve is needed to master this technique [6].

Light-guided injection seems to be preclinical stage, and there has been no clinical study for human so far. Several studies with ex-vivo animal model or cadaver showed that guidance of light at the tip of injection needle can improve the accuracy of percutaneous needle localization in the larynx (Fig. 13.1). On contrast to the previous blind technique which depends on the operator's touch sensation on the internal laryngeal structures, this technique directly visualizes the location of needle tip in the larynx. This helps not only the operator, especially the novice, to locate the needle tip at the appropriate site, but also the trainees (residents or fellows) to learn the needle passage and location during the entire procedure of injection laryngoplasty [7].

13.3 Ultrasound Guided Injection

Ultrasound as guiding purposes for laryngeal procedure (Fig. 13.2) is used to increase the accuracy of diagnosis and treatment and help minimize damage to surrounding tissues when invasive procedures are performed. Ultrasound-guided needle aspiration (e.g., abscess and cyst) is the same as in other areas, while unique utilization in the larynx is typical of laryngeal injection and laryngeal electromyography.

There has been no report with regard to the injection laryngoplasty exclusively depending on the ultrasound without endoscope. Ng et al. reported a technique of combined ultrasound/endoscopic assisted transcutaneous transcartilage vocal cord injection [8]. Although they showed that the use of ultrasound in aiding transcutaneous transcartilaginous vocal cord injection is safe and feasible, ultrasound is difficult to apply when the thyroid cartilage is thick and heavily calcified. In addition, in other than transcartilaginous approach, ultrasound cannot visualize the needle passage from skin to injection site. Relative lower resolution than endoscope and blurry mucosal margin are hurdles for the successful injection.

13.4 Others

Some patients may be intolerable to the laryngeal injection procedure under local anesthesia. While laryngeal injection under general anesthesia can be another option, conventional endotracheal tube may hinder surgical view and interfere with determining the exact vocal fold position in case of injection laryngoplasty. Mayerhoff et al. reported that injection laryngoplasty using supraglottic airway can be feasible [9]. Advantages include maintenance of spontaneous ventilation without paralysis, no neck

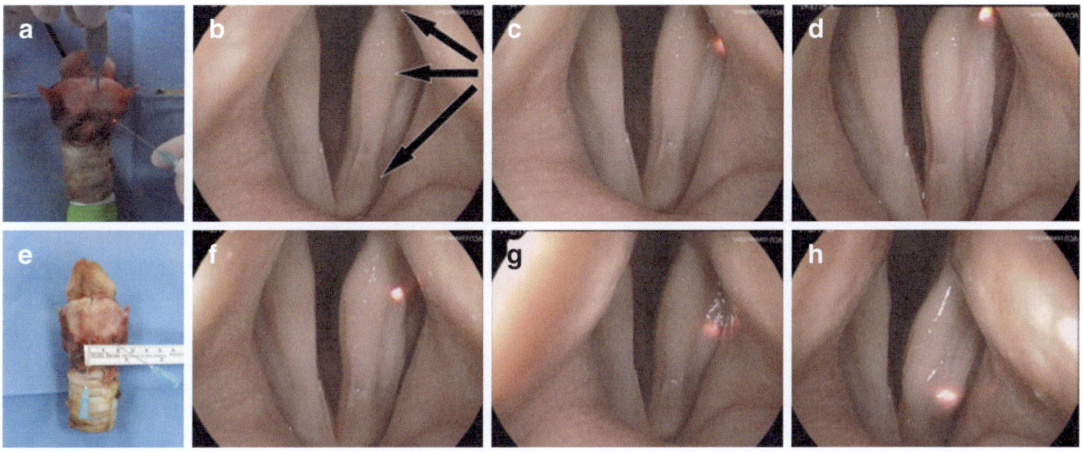

Fig. 13.1 To simulate VFI at the insertion points that are relatively far lateral compared to the conventional insertion point, we performed VFI from insertion points 17 mm from the midline, which is lateral to the conventional point. (**a**) The needle insertion at the point 17 mm from the midline in the cadaveric canine model, simulating the setting of office-based VFI. (**e**) The midline and the insertion point (17 mm) are indicated with the two needles in the canine larynx. (**b**) The imaginary routes of the needle tip are indicated by the black arrow. (**c**, **d**, **f**–**h**) When the injector was introduced at the insertion point 17 mm from the midline, the light of needle tip was initially identified at the lateral and posterior parts of vocal fold (**c**). Different from the conventional (10 mm) and the medial (3 mm) insertion points, the needle could be introduced into the vocal fold in various directions of posteromedial (**d**), medial (**f**), and anteromedial (**g**, **h**) under light guidance. The needle tip could be positioned at the intended point of the left vocal fold, as indicated by the light. *VFI* vocal fold injection. *(figures from prof. Wonjae Cha)*

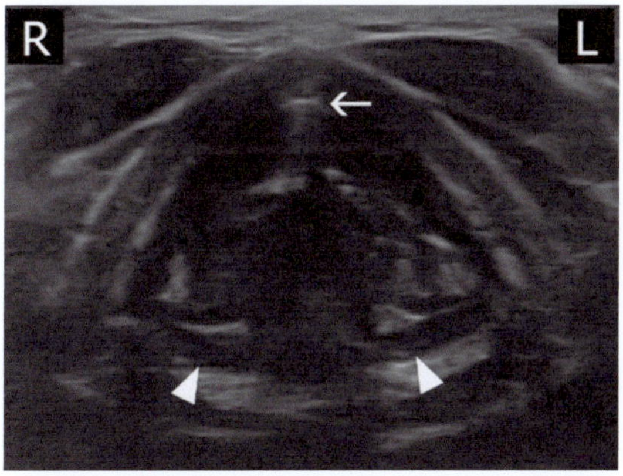

Fig. 13.2 Normal ultrasound anatomy of larynx. Anterior commissure is hyperechoic in ultrasound (arrow). Internal and external laryngeal muscles are generally hypoechoic in ultrasound. Arytenoid cartilage is generally hyperechoic when it is less ossified, while hypoechoic when more ossified. The false vocal fold is hyperechoic compared to the true vocal fold

extension, improved patient tolerance, and accommodation of difficult anatomy. Although there are disadvantages, such as increased time and cost related to the operating room, supraglottic airway permits injection laryngoplasty in previously ineligible patients. Grant et al. reported that video laryngoscope and laryngeal injector can be another option for patients with intravenous sedation and be performed without interference of endotracheal tube [10].

Key Learning Points:

- Trans-nasal approach is advantageous for those with strong gag reflex, while inability to separate the endoscopic view and angle of injection needle is disadvantage.
- Light-guided injection technique is still preclinical stage, while it can be useful in clinical setting especially for the novice and trainee to localize the correct needle tip during the procedure.
- Although ultrasound enables to visualize the larynx without endoscope through oral or nasal cavity, low resolution and uncertainty of vocal fold mucosal margin are hurdles to overcome.

References

1. Trask DK, Shellenberger DL, Hoffman HT. Transnasal, endoscopic vocal fold augmentation. Laryngoscope. 2005;115:2262–5.
2. Hamdan AL, Ziade G, Jaffal H, Skaff G. Transnasal injection Laryngoplasty. Ann Oto Rhinol Laryn. 2015;124:474–9.
3. Maccarini AR, Stacchini M, Mozzanica F, et al. Efficacy of trans-nasal fiberendoscopic injection laryngoplasty with centrifuged autologous fat in the treatment of glottic insufficiency due to unilateral vocal fold paralysis. Acta Otorhinolaryngo. 2018;38:204–13.
4. Joseph EB, Christopher PG, Jodie EMG, Maria PM, Anh H, Thomas LC. Injectable silk protein microparticle-based fillers: a novel material for potential use in Glottic insufficiency. J Voice. 2019;33:773–80.
5. Chi-Te W, Mei-Shu L, Li-Jen L, Wu-Chia L, Po-Wen C. Transnasal endoscopic steroid injection: a practical and effective alternative treatment for benign vocal fold disorders. Laryngoscope. 2013;123:1464–8.
6. Hoffman HT, Dailey SH, Bock JM, Thibeault SL, McCulloch TM. Transillumination for needle localization in the larynx. Laryngoscope. 2015;125:2341–8.
7. Cha W, Ro JH, Yang SCet al. Real-time light-guided vocal fold injection: ex vivo feasibility study in a canine model. Laryngoscope 2019; 129:935–942.
8. Ng SK, Yuen HY, van Hasselt CA, Ahuja A. Combined ultrasound/endoscopy-assisted vocal fold injection for unilateral vocal cord paralysis: a case series. Eur Radiol. 2012;22:1110–3.
9. Mayerhoff RM, Kuo C, Meyer T. A novel approach to the challenging injection Laryngoplasty. Ann Oto Rhinol Laryn. 2016;125:415–20.
10. Grant NN, Holliday MA, Lima R. Use of the video-laryngoscope (GlideScope) in vocal fold injection medialization. Laryngoscope. 2014;124:2136–8.

Part IV

Postoperative Considerations

14 Post-Injection Care and Complication Management

Young-Ik Son

Abstract

Injection laryngoplasty is generally considered a safe procedure. However, it should be used with full understanding of the potential serious adverse reactions such as systemic hypersensitivity reaction, airway compromise, granuloma formation, and necrosis of the vocal fold. A wide range of side effects has been reported, which include early onset erythema, bruising, edema, and irritation at the injection site. Delayed effects include persistent erythema, edema, nodule formation, and implant migration. During the learning curve, suboptimal voice outcome secondary to superficial injection or over-injection is not an infrequent complication. Even for experienced surgeons, failure of office-based injection may happen, which is secondary to difficult anatomy or poor patient tolerance. There are no gold-standard guidelines regarding the post-injection care including duration of close observation, medications, and voice rest after injection laryngoplasty. In general, checking perioperative vital signs and monitoring respiratory distress symptoms are recommended for more than an hour.

Y.-I. Son (✉)
Department of Otorhinolaryngology - Head and Neck Surgery, Samsung Medical Center, Sungkyunkwan University School of Medicine, Seoul, South Korea
e-mail: yison@skku.edu

Keywords

Postoperative management · Complications Failure · Suboptimal injection

14.1 Complication Management

14.1.1 Introduction

Bruening performed the first injection laryngoplasty with paraffin in 1911. Since that time, various injectable substances have been used for injection laryngoplasty to treat glottic insufficiency. Temporary materials include carboxymethylcellulose (Radiesse Voice Gel; BioForm Medical, Franksville, Wisconsin), hyaluronic acid gel (Restylane; Q-Med Scandinavia, Princeton, Virginia; Hylaform; Q-Med, Uppsala, Sweden), micronized collagen (Cymetra; LifeCell Corporation, Bridgewater, New Jersey), bovine collagen (Zyplast; Advanced Dermatology PC, New York, New York), and bovine gelatin (Gelfoam; Pfizer, New York, New York; Surgifoam; Ethicon, Centreville, Virginia). Long lasting materials include calcium hydroxylapatite (Radiesse Voice; BioForm Medical), ArteSense (European Medical Contract Manufacturing B.V., Nijmegen, The Netherlands), autologous fat, and, of historic importance, polytetrafluoroethylene (PTFE) paste (Teflon; Dupont, Wilmington, Delaware) [1, 2]. Each of these substances has demonstrated

© Springer Nature Singapore Pte Ltd. 2021
B.-J. Lee et al. (eds.), *Vocal Fold Injection*, https://doi.org/10.1007/978-981-16-3303-4_14

limitations, such as hypersensitivity, migration from the injection site, inflammation, and granuloma formation [3]. The use of Teflon has decreased markedly after the identification of long-term complications such as foreign body reactions, granuloma formation, and lymphatic migration of PTFE particles [4].

Despite injection laryngoplasty is generally considered a safe procedure, a wide range of side effects can occur. Therefore, physicians who perform vocal fold injections with these materials should be aware of the potential complications. Early onset complications are erythema, bruising, edema, and irritation at the injection site. Delayed effects include persistent erythema, edema, nodule formation, and implant migration [5]. The more serious side effects are systemic hypersensitivity reaction, airway compromise with hematoma, granuloma formation, laryngeal abscess, ulceration, and necrosis of the vocal fold. During the learning curve, suboptimal voice outcomes secondary to superficial injection or over-injection are not infrequent complication [6]. Even for experienced surgeons, failure of office-based injection may happen, which is secondary to difficult anatomy or poor patient tolerance [7].

14.1.2 Calcium Hydroxlyapatite (CaHA)

De Fatta et al. reported 19 complications out of 22 vocal fold injections with CaHA. Ten major complications included adynamic mucosa, a severely decreased wave, and granulomas affecting the vibratory margin. Nine minor complications included tissue inflammation marked by edema, erythema, and mild-to-moderate mucosal wave restriction and hypervascularity [3]. Cohen et al. reported a case of severe systemic reaction consisted of diffuse itching, hives, edematous face and eyelids, and voice changes indicating glottic edema. The reaction occurred within 30 min of the procedure [8]. A case of pulmonary embolism was reported after percutaneous injection of CaHA [9].

Lee et al. reported a single physician's experiences of 955 office-based CaHA injection laryngoplasty using the cricothyroid approach; Five cases were failed (0.5%), superficial injection occurred in eight cases (0.8%), acute and delayed onset dyspnea was observed in three (0.3%) and two (0.2%) cases, respectively. Most complications recorded in their study were intraprocedural complications, which were related to technical problems rather than CaHA itself. Most of the complications primarily occurred early in the learning curve [6].

Chheda et al. studied the institutional rates of suboptimal injection at four Voice and Swallowing centers, which ranged from 0.4 to 0.9%. If a superficial injection has been identified, microflap endoscopic techniques should be performed to preserve vibratory function. For cases of over medialization, a limited cordotomy provided excellent access to the material [10]. Recognition of superficially injected or overaugmented vocal folds at the time of initial injection is the optimal time to treat and correct the problem. However, even delayed recognition of problems can usually be managed with satisfactory outcomes by careful removal of CaHA [11].

14.1.3 Collagen; Cymetra, Zyplast

Concerns about hypersensitivity reactions to bovine antigens (Zyplast) in 3% of patients led to the development of cadaveric collagen derived from acellular micronized dermis (Cymetra). However, Luu et al. reported that there were no allergic complications in 845 patients who did not undergo skin hypersensitivity testing before injection laryngoplasty with Zyplast [12]. Reported complications of Cymetra injections were intralaryngeal abscess, [13] decreased mucosal wave after superficial injection, [14] migration from the vocal fold to the medial wall of the pyriform sinus [4]. Tan et al. reported their 10-year experience with 381 Cymetra injections in 344 patients. There were four complications for 381 injections (1.05%); postoperative stridor, infection at the injection site, and contact granuloma secondary to over-injection. Five patients (1.31%) experienced injection failure due to technical issues [15].

14.1.4 Hyaluronic Acid (Restylane)

Laryngeal reactions to Restylane are very rare. However, there were several reports of airway compromise, which consisted of severe edema at the injection site of the vocal fold, false vocal fold, and aryepiglottic fold [5, 16, 17]. Hamdan el al. reported three cases (4.7%) of adverse reaction after injection laryngoplasty with hyaluronic acid in 63 patients. They complained progressive shortness of breath, dysphagia, and globus sensation. Flexible laryngoscopy revealed edema extending to the aryepiglottic fold and redness of the true and false vocal folds [18].

There are three possible mechanisms for the adverse reactions to hyaluronic acid. First is allergic or local hypersensitivity reaction, with the sensitivity being attributed to the fermenting bacteria (streptococci) in the manufacturing process [18]. Second is an acute infection of bacterial origin that causes inflammation with fluctuant and erythematous nodules. A third possible theory is ischemic event secondary to vascular compression or occlusion by the injected material [5, 17].

Halderman et al. reported their experiences of office-based injections with Restylane. Of 82 injections in 64 patients, a total of five adverse events (6.1%) were documented; superficial injection into the subepithelial plane, atrial fibrillation at the end of procedure, edema of the false and true vocal folds ipsilateral to the injection, and a hematoma of the arytenoid on a patient of Coumadin therapy [16].

14.1.5 Special Consideration

Dang et al. reported that there was no observed difference in bleeding complications between patients who were continued on antiplatelet or anticoagulation treatment versus those whose therapy was withheld [19].

However, Sato et al. observed three cases (6.4%) of bleeding in patients who were on antithrombotic drugs (47 injections). Fortunately, no patients exhibited airway narrowing or dyspnea [20]. Halderman et al. reported a case of hematoma at the arytenoid on a patient of Coumadin therapy [16].

Mathison et al. reported a slightly higher complication rate (odds ratio, 2.9) in the awake patient than the asleep patient [21]. In contrast, Kelly et al. demonstrated a low complication rate (2.3%, 4 out of 174 procedures) of bilateral injections in the office-based, awake setting [7]. Chheda el al. emphasized that less experienced surgeons should perform injection in the operating room under controlled general anesthetic conditions to minimize the potential for suboptimal placement [10].

14.2 Post-Injection Care

There are no standard guidelines regarding the perioperative management including duration of close observation, medications, and voice rest after injection laryngoplasty.

Halderman et al. checked vital signs before and after each injection. They monitored patients for variable periods until the patients were comfortable leaving the clinic or simply remained in their hospital bed with routine nursing care [16]. My patients are usually observed for about 2 hours in a recovery room while checking their vital signs and monitoring symptoms related with respiratory distress. They can talk and have some food since that time [22]. Lee et al. allowed the patients to leave after 1 h of observation at the outpatient clinic; they were instructed to avoid talking until the next day and prescribed oral analgesics that could be taken when required [6]. Hamdan et al. recommended close observation of patients for a period of 24 h while monitoring symptoms such as lump sensation in the throat, dysphagia, and/or shortness of breath [18].

DeFatta et al. tried to minimize postoperative cough, vomiting, upper respiratory infection, and laryngopharyngeal reflux, which could possibly contribute to inflammation and even implant migration. Patients diagnosed with LPR preoperatively were treated with a proton pump inhibitor twice daily and an H2 blocker at bedtime.

Seven days of voice rest was prescribed after vocal fold injection to help optimize implant stability [3].

Key Learning Points:

- Although injection laryngoplasty is generally considered a safe procedure, it should be used with full understanding of the potential serious adverse reactions as well as the risk of diverse minor complications.
- During the learning curve, suboptimal voice outcomes secondary to superficial injection or over-injection are not rare complication.
- Even for experienced surgeons, failure of office-based injection may happen, which is secondary to difficult anatomy or poor patient tolerance.
- Checking vital signs and monitoring respiratory distress symptoms are recommended for more than an hour after injection laryngoplasty.

References

1. Vachha BA, Ginat DT, Mallur P, Cunnane M, Moonis G. "finding a voice": imaging features after Phonosurgical procedures for vocal fold paralysis. AJNR Am J Neuroradiol. 2016;37(9):1574–80. Epub 2016/05/14. eng
2. Choi N, Jin H, Kim HJ, Son YI. Early injection Laryngoplasty with a long-lasting material in patients with potentially recoverable unilateral vocal fold paralysis. Clin Exp Otorhinolaryngol. 2019;12(4):427–32.
3. DeFatta RA, Chowdhury FR, Sataloff RT. Complications of injection laryngoplasty using calcium hydroxylapatite. J Voice. 2012;26(5):614–8. Epub 2011/11/08. eng
4. Bock JM, Lee JH, Robinson RA, Hoffman HT. Migration of Cymetra after vocal fold injection for laryngeal paralysis. Laryngoscope. 2007;117(12):2251–4. Epub 2007/10/03. eng
5. Shamanna SG, Bosch JD. Injection laryngoplasty: a serious reaction to hyaluronic acid. J Otolaryngol Head Neck Surg. 2011;40(5):E39–42. Epub 2012/03/17. eng.
6. Lee M, Lee DY, Kwon TK. Safety of office-based percutaneous injection laryngoplasty with calcium hydroxylapatite. Laryngoscope. 2019;129(10):2361–5. Epub 2019/02/14. eng
7. Kelly Z, Patel AK, Klein AM. Evaluating safety of awake, bilateral injection Laryngoplasty for bilateral vocal fold atrophy. J Voice. 2020;7. Epub 2020/03/12. eng
8. Cohen JC, Reisacher W, Malone M, Sulica L. Severe systemic reaction from calcium hydroxylapatite vocal fold filler. Laryngoscope. 2013;123(9):2237–9. Epub 2013/07/04. eng
9. Won SJ, Woo SH. Calcium Hydroxylapatite pulmonary embolism after percutaneous injection Laryngoplasty. Yonsei Med J. 2017;58(6):1245–8. Epub 2017/10/20. eng
10. Chheda NN, Rosen CA, Belafsky PC, Simpson CB, Postma GN. Revision laryngeal surgery for the suboptimal injection of calcium hydroxylapatite. Laryngoscope. 2008;118(12):2260–3. Epub 2008/11/26. eng
11. Ting JY, Patel R, Halum SL. Managing voice impairment after injection laryngoplasty. J Voice. 2012;26(6):797–800. Epub 2012/05/29. eng
12. Luu Q, Tsai V, Mangunta V, Berke GS, Chhetri DK. Safety of percutaneous injection of bovine dermal crosslinked collagen for glottic insufficiency. Otolaryngol Head Neck Surg. 2007;136(3):445–9. Epub 2007/02/27. eng
13. Zapanta PE, Bielamowicz SA. Laryngeal abscess after injection laryngoplasty with micronized AlloDerm. Laryngoscope. 2004;114(9):1522–4. Epub 2004/10/12. eng
14. Anderson TD, Sataloff RT. Complications of collagen injection of the vocal fold: report of several unusual cases and review of the literature. J Voice. 2004;18(3):392–7. Epub 2004/08/28. eng
15. Tan M, Woo P. Injection laryngoplasty with micronized dermis: a 10-year experience with 381 injections in 344 patients. Laryngoscope. 2010;120(12):2460–6. Epub 2010/10/26. eng
16. Halderman AA, Bryson PC, Benninger MS, Chota R. Safety and length of benefit of restylane for office-based injection medialization-a retrospective review of one institution's experience. J Voice. 2014;28(5):631–5. Epub 2014/02/18. eng
17. Traboulsi H, El Natout T, Skaff G, Hamdan AL. Adverse reaction to hyaluronic acid injection laryngoplasty: a case report. J Voice. 2017;31(2):245.e1-.e2. Epub 2016/10/26. eng.
18. Hamdan AL, Khalifee E. Adverse reaction to Restylane: a review of 63 cases of injection Laryngoplasty. Ear Nose Throat J. 2019;98(4):212–6. Epub 2019/03/28. eng
19. Dang JH, Liou NE, Ongkasuwan J. Anticoagulation and antiplatelet therapy in awake transcervical injection laryngoplasty. Laryngoscope. 2017;127(8):1850–4. Epub 2017/03/09. eng

20. Sato T, Nito T, Ueha R, Goto T, Yamasoba T. Investigation of the safety of injection Laryngoplasty under antithrombotic therapy. ORL. 2019;81(4):215–23. Epub 2019/07/29. eng
21. Mathison CC, Villari CR, Klein AM, Johns MM 3rd. Comparison of outcomes and complications between awake and asleep injection laryngoplasty: a case-control study. Laryngoscope. 2009;119(7):1417–23. Epub 2009/06/10. eng
22. Choi N, Won S, Jin H, Kim HJ, Park W, Son YI. Additional injection laryngoplasty for patients with unilateral vocal fold paralysis. Laryngoscope. 2020;130(12):2863–8.

Perioperative Voice Therapy 15

Alexandra Mechler-Hickson and Susan L. Thibeault

Abstract

Voice therapy should be a component of treatment for any dysphonic patient. Indirect therapy centered around voice hygiene and patient education, as well as direct therapy that intervenes on the physiology of phonation, are both important to include as treatment options. Voice therapy has been studied in the treatment of a variety of conditions that may also include vocal fold injection as part of their treatment, including benign vocal fold lesions, vocal fold paralysis, presbyphonia, and laryngeal tremor. There is evidence of patient benefit with even one session of preoperative voice therapy, and a variety of studies to support the use of postoperative therapy as well. Content, timing, and duration of voice therapy has not been standardized, and in the absence of this should be decided between the individual patient and their speech-language pathologist.

Keywords

Voice therapy · Speech therapy · Behavioral Perioperative · Postoperative · Preoperative

A. Mechler-Hickson · S. L. Thibeault (✉)
Division of Otolaryngology Head and Neck Surgery, Department of Surgery, University of Wisconsin-Madison, Madison, WI, USA
e-mail: thibeaul@surgery.wisc.edu

15.1 Introduction

Voice therapy is an important component of dysphonia management, both as primary and adjunctive therapy. Per the 2018 American Academy of Otolaryngology—Head and Neck Surgery clinical practice guidelines for dysphonia, voice therapy may be incorporated as a component of any surgical dysphonia treatment, and a basic understanding of its strengths is thus of use to any practicing laryngologist [1]. In this chapter, we will first briefly define the scope of voice therapy services and measures of its success, then discuss the evidence for the use of voice therapy in a variety of voice conditions amenable to procedural intervention. We will additionally incorporate a discussion on the ideal duration and timing of voice therapy, as well as patient characteristics associated with greater treatment benefit.

15.2 Prior to Speech-Language Pathology Involvement

Diagnostic laryngoscopy with stroboscopy should be performed prior to patient referral to a speech-language pathologist (SLP) for voice therapy and all results should be communicated with the SLP if they are not part of the evaluative team [1, 2]. Establishing an organic or functional diagnosis prior to referral aids in voice therapy planning and excludes patients with lesions

© Springer Nature Singapore Pte Ltd. 2021

B.-J. Lee et al. (eds.), *Vocal Fold Injection*, https://doi.org/10.1007/978-981-16-3303-4_15

generally inappropriate for treatment with voice therapy, such as laryngeal malignancy [1, 3–5].

15.3 Indirect and Direct Voice Therapy

When considering different voice therapy techniques, it is useful to categorize them into indirect and direct interventions. Indirect interventions center around changing the behavioral, psychological, and environmental factors that help both precipitate and maintain abnormal voicing [6, 7]. These include provision of knowledge regarding proper voice use, as well as identification and mitigation of voice stressors in the patient's life [6, 8, 9]. SLPs may review principles of vocal fold health, recommend optimized management of allergy and laryngopharyngeal reflux symptoms, counsel regarding avoidance of phonotraumatic voice use, and assess psychological factors that may impact voicing as a part of this treatment course.

Alternatively, direct interventions involve modification of voicing physiology. These may be grouped into alterations in several categories, including: motor execution of voicing, response to somatosensory input and response to auditory input [6, 8, 9]. Tools utilized to this end are diverse, and may include exercises such as pitch and loudness modification, respiratory coordination and support of voicing, neck, orofacial and postural modifications, as well as adjustments made based on patient nociception [6].

There is evidence to suggest that both indirect and direct therapy may play a role in vocal rehabilitation, but there has been no definitive conclusion as to how much of each is most effective. A 2008 meta-analysis found that a combination of both direct and indirect voice therapy was effective at improving vocal functioning in those with functional dysphonia [10]. In a randomized control trial by MacKenzie et al., a combination of the two methods produced voice improvement based on a self-reported voice profile questionnaire as well as measurement of shimmer [11]. Similarly, Carding et al. report that 93% of patients with nonorganic dysphonia treated with a combination of indirect and direct therapies showed significant improvement in voice quality [7]. In a randomized control trial by Gilivan-Murphy et al., a combination of vocal function exercises and voice hygiene education in teachers with self-reported voice problems demonstrated significant voice improvement as measured by the Voice Symptom Severity Scale [12].

Comparison of the two types of intervention is made difficult by lack of alternative treatment for control groups and an absence of standardized treatment protocols, particularly between different voice conditions (ex. muscle tension dysphonia, Parkinson-related voice therapy, laryngeal nerve paralysis/paresis, vocal fold lesions). However, there is some literature demonstrating benefit of direct voice therapy alone. A systematic review by Speyer et al. in 2008 found insufficient evidence to draw strong conclusions but did note that direct voice therapy tended to be more effective than indirect interventions alone [13, 14]. More recently, a 2017 review of voice therapy did demonstrate superiority by self-reported and objective voice measurements of interventions involving direct voice therapy [15], including in women with benign phonotraumatic vocal fold lesions [16], in 42 patients that had a functional alteration in voice function or benign laryngeal lesions [17] and 20 patients primarily being treated for muscle tension dysphonia [18]. Interestingly, in a 2014 study eliciting patient preferences amongst vocal hygiene interventions and direct voice therapy, patients reported direct voice therapy exercises as what they considered most useful [19]. This preference is perhaps reflected in the proportion of time during appointments dedicated to direct vs. indirect voice therapy. Gartner-Schmidt et al. report that direct voice therapy comprised upwards of 75% of the treatment time in SLP appointments they reviewed [20].

Despite literature supporting the use of direct over indirect voice therapy, there is also reported benefit with the exclusive use of indirect methods. Carding et al. found that in their study of patients with nonorganic dysphonia, 46% of patients who received exclusively indirect voice therapy experienced significant change in voice quality [7]. In a 1994 study by Chan, kindergarten teachers who underwent a voice hygiene intervention showed both acoustic and electroglottic improvement of voice versus those who did not [21]. Yun et al. 2007 demonstrated a decrease in vocal fold polyp size in 20% of patients treated with voice hygiene therapy alone [22], and a separate study from the same year showed greater patient benefit in both vocal characteristics and voice knowledge following indirect (versus direct) voice therapy [23]. In the perioperative population in particular, Koufman and Blalock noted that postoperative dysphonia was closely associated with lack of vocal hygiene counseling or adherence to hygiene recommendations [24, 25].

Overall, there is no clear optimal proportion of direct and indirect voice therapy, as both strategies have been shown to offer some benefit and studies often do not completely describe the voice therapy they perform. Our recommendation at this time is for voice therapy content to be individualized to each patient based on SLP recommendations and patient willingness to participate in and adhere to each type of intervention. In the perioperative period, it may be universally useful to include education as to expected changes in voice following procedures, how long this will be expected to last and what hygiene measures should be undertaken to avoid recurrent or persistent dysphonia. Additionally, direct interventions may include exercises to both reduce compensatory hyperfunction that could interfere with an optimal surgical result and minimize vocal fold inflammation from phonotrauma.

15.4 Outcome Metrics in Voice Therapy

As alluded to previously, there are a diverse array of outcome measures related to voice therapy, including self-reported voice improvement, voice quality on physical examination, acoustic and aerodynamic measures, and direct laryngeal examination [26]. While these measures are all commonly reported in the literature, they do not necessarily display a direct correlation to one another, at times making meaningful comparison between studies challenging [15, 27–29].

15.5 Benign Vocal Fold Lesions

Treatment of benign vocal fold lesions (BVFLs), including vocal fold polyps, nodules, cysts, and other lesions [30], may all incorporate voice therapy as a component of their treatment [1, 19, 31]. This is done with the intention of minimizing vocal behaviors that would increase mechanical stress at the mid-membranous vocal fold [31]. In particular, voice therapy for benign vocal fold lesions centers around patient education, attempts to change maladaptive voice behaviors and modify environmental factors which may allow for persistence of the lesion [32]. However, direct therapy remains an important component as well: in one study of patient perceptions of voice therapy, those with benign vocal fold lesions reported finding direct interventions particularly useful [19].

In patients with vocal fold nodules, both direct and indirect voice therapy is generally approached as a primary treatment modality [33–35]. A recent review of voice therapy in vocal fold nodules was conducted by Mansuri et al. in 2018. They found that indirect therapy interventions were used in addition to a variety of direct voice therapies such as reciprocal inhibition, optimal pitch, the Smith Accent Method, tongue trill, Lessac-Madsen Resonant Voice Therapy and Vocal Function Exercises. In all included studies, voice therapy did provide a range of benefits, including improved voice quality, decrease in nodule size or resolution of vocal fold nodules [36]. Interestingly, an investigation by Murry and Woodson cited in this review compared three treatment groups: group one received voice therapy without otolaryngologist consultation, group two was referred to voice therapy following surgical nodule excision, and group three had a combined evaluation from speech-language pathology and otolaryngology but ultimately underwent primary voice therapy. Group three exhibited the greatest voice improvement as determined by perceptual rating of voice recordings [37]. In the perioperative period, voice therapy may be important for treatment of vocal fold nodules, with one study of 62 patients showing a correlation between absence of postoperative voice therapy and nodule recurrence [38].

Voice therapy is less commonly relied upon in patients with vocal fold polyps and cysts, but there is some evidence for its use as a primary treatment and it is commonly employed as an adjunct [31, 33, 35, 39–41]. In a study of over 600 patients with polyps that compared voice therapy and medication with surgery, polyps resolved in almost 10% of patients who received conservative measures [42]. Other studies similarly found that in some patients, a course of voice therapy could obviate the need for subsequent phonosurgery in patients with vocal fold polyps [22, 43–46]. In a 2017 study by Barillari et al., in 140 patients with polyps there was no significant difference in outcome between groups sorted to treatment by standard voice therapy combined with phonosurgery and a "voice therapy expulsion" protocol, suggesting that the expulsion protocol could be utilized as primary treatment. However, it is worth noting that in this study those who underwent "standard" voice therapy (with both indirect and direct components) had only non-significant improvement in self-reported voice measures following conservative intervention. All 70 of the patients in this group progressed to phonosurgery, the implication being that standard voice therapy alone was insufficient treatment [47].

Perioperatively, a 2018 study by Sahin et al. found that in treatment of vocal fold polyps, voice therapy alone was unfavorable when compared to phonosurgery alone, but that voice therapy with phonosurgery demonstrated a greater improvement in self-rated and perceptual characteristics than either intervention in isolation [48]. Similarly, Petrovic-Lazic et al. suggest that postoperative voice therapy can help to further improve voice following polyp excision in both perceptual characteristics and acoustic measures [49]. Lin et al. report that patients who received postoperative voice training had improved voice on self-rated, perceptual, and acoustic measurements, leading to better vocal rehabilitation [50]. In multiple other studies, adjunctive postoperative voice therapy was also associated with improvement in self-reported measures such as the Voice Handicap Index, with less conclusive results in acoustic and aerodynamic measurements [51, 52].

Vocal fold cysts are also not thought to be as amenable to primary treatment with voice therapy as a definitive solution [33, 34]. However, conservative intervention, of which voice therapy is one option, may still help to improve voicing. In a study by Cohen et al., 60% of patients with vocal fold cysts who received voice therapy reported voice improvement at their final follow-up appointment, defined as the ability to meet their daily voice needs most of the time [44]. In many cases postoperative voice therapy is utilized as an adjunct for patients with vocal fold cysts [34], but its benefits have not been evaluated to the same extent as other benign lesions. In a 2018 retrospective review of 24 patients who underwent vocal fold cyst excision, patients reported improvement in their voice regardless of the addition of voice therapy following the procedure: there was no significant difference in change in Voice Handicap Index between the two groups [53].

Other benign vocal fold lesions, such as Reinke's edema and vocal fold granuloma, may also incorporate voice therapy as part of their treatment. Schindler et al. included patients with Reinke's edema in prospective cohort study of the effect of voice therapy on BVFLs, and noted that in particular patients with Reinke's edema had improved voice quality by perceptual characteristics after voice therapy [31]. In a study of 10 patients who underwent a voice therapy program for reflux-related vocal process granuloma, the 8 patients who completed the program experienced improvement or complete resolution of their pathology [54]. Ylitalo and Hammarberg also investigated the effect of voice therapy on patients with laryngeal granuloma, and found that voice therapy improved patient fundamental frequency [55].

Considering BVFLs more broadly, there is additional support for the use of perioperative voice therapy. In 2017, Tang and Thibeault conducted a retrospective review to study the ideal timing of perioperative therapy for those with benign lesions. They found that groups who received both preoperative and postoperative therapy as well as those who had postoperative therapy alone had improvement in their Voice Handicap Index scores. However, only those who had received preoperative interventions exhibited a statistically significant change in these self-reported voice outcomes.

It should be noted that throughout literature discussing voice therapy for BVFLs, including the perioperative period, the level of evidence is persistently low and an area of opportunity for future research [33, 40, 56]. In Mansuri et al.'s review of nodules as well as a Cochrane review comparing voice therapy and phonosurgical intervention for nodules, authors recommended further investigation and stated that higher quality evidence was needed to draw strong conclusions [36, 57]. Similarly, an overarching systematic review of voice therapy for functional, organic, and neurological voice disorders noted that while high-quality evidence existed for the efficacy of voice therapy in the general treatment of vocal fold nodules, the literature was less definitive regarding other BVFLs [32].

15.6 Vocal Fold Paralysis

Vocal fold paresis and paralysis may be treated with a combination of voice therapy and procedural intervention depending on examination findings and patient preferences [58]. There are a variety of studies showing voice improvement following primary voice therapy in patients with vocal fold paresis or paralysis based on a variety of measures, including self-reported [3, 59–63], perceptual [59–64], acoustic [59–61, 63, 65], and aerodynamic testing [61, 64]. Recent reviews of the use of voice therapy in vocal fold paralysis note that while overall these studies demonstrate a positive effect, there is little robust evidence to make conclusions about its overall efficacy or ideal treatment protocol [32, 66].

Data on the perioperative use of voice therapy in vocal fold paralysis patients is limited. In Heuer et al. 1997, patients with recurrent laryngeal nerve paralysis were treated with voice therapy and were subsequently offered surgical intervention if they did not feel their voice was adequately improved. Sixty-eight percent of female patients and 64% of male patients improved sufficiently with voice therapy alone, eliminating the need for surgery. The authors noted that by objective measures, the group that received both voice therapy and surgery had greater voice improvement, but that by satisfaction with voice outcome the groups were equivalent [67].

15.7 Presbyphonia

Presbyphonia is a condition treated with voice therapy to improve breathing patterns, muscle tension and glottal closure for optimization of phonation [68]. Surgical intervention may also be considered if voice therapy is insufficient, either via injection augmentation or thyroplasty [69]. Indirect and direct voice therapy interventions may be used: the largest body of literature evaluating primary voice therapy in this population focuses on different direct interventions, which have been shown to provide benefit to patients through both subjective and objective measures [70–77].

The perioperative effect of voice therapy in this condition is something that has not been well-elucidated to date, and is an area of opportunity for investigation [69]. In one retrospective study by Garter-Schmidt and Rosen, 86 patients receiving treatment for vocal fold atrophy were reviewed, with notable groups being those who ultimately elected for no treatment (31%), had voice therapy alone (44%), had surgery alone (15%), and those who had voice therapy followed by surgery (9%). Treatment success, defined as a reduction in Voice Handicap Index of greater than five following the intervention, was achieved in 36% of patients receiving voice therapy alone, 56% after surgery alone, and in 17% of patients following a combination of the two. It should be noted that the sample size for groups including surgical intervention were low (9 patients had surgery alone, 8 patients had this and voice therapy) and not all patients had a complete data set, making drawing strong conclusions from this study difficult [78].

Postoperatively, Tanner et al. describe the use of voice therapy in a case of vocal fold bowing in elderly monozygotic twins. Both twins underwent bilateral Hylaform-medialization procedures with temporally limited, modest voice improvements afterwards. Following this, both patients had a 3-month course of direct voice therapy, after which time they exhibited improvement based on Voice Handicap Index scores and on glottal closure configuration during endoscopic examination despite some persistent dysphonia [79].

15.8 Laryngeal Dystonia

Laryngeal dystonia is a group of disorders including spasmodic dysphonia, essential voice tremor and the rigid, hypokinetic dysphonia associated with Parkinson's disease. Treatment of these disorders, similarly to those discussed previously, may be multimodal.

Spasmodic dysphonia is a hyperkinetic disorder for which the standard treatment is typically Botulinum toxin injection or other procedural or medical intervention [80, 81]. Voice therapy is typically thought to have less of a role when compared to other disorders, with sparse evidence for symptomatic improvement with direct voice therapy [82]. There is additionally limited evidence for the use of periprocedural voice therapy. A 1995 study by Murry and Woodson compared patients treated with a combined-modality approach of botulinum toxin injection and post-injection direct voice therapy with those who received only botulinum toxin injections. The multimodal treatment group, in whom direct voice therapy attempted to regulate both extrinsic muscle hyperfunction and breathing abnormalities with phonation, experienced a statistically significant greater average duration between botulinum toxin injections (average 27.4 weeks in the voice therapy group vs. 14.9 weeks in the injection-only group). They also exhibited greater improvement of acoustic and aerodynamic voice parameters, and it was concluded that voice therapy could be a useful adjunct to injection [83]. Additionally, a 2009 study comparing voice rest following vocal fold injection for spasmodic dysphonia with voice exercise found that injection cycles incorporating immediate postprocedural voice therapy may be more efficacious based on improved patient satisfaction even with decreased doses of botulinum toxin [84]. In contrast to these results, Silverman et al. also compared patients who received botulinum toxin injections to those receiving injections as well as voice therapy, and also compared a group receiving injections and sham voice therapy. Their investigation did not find any significant difference between groups in terms of treatment duration, or acoustic or aerodynamic measures [85]. Thus, the role of periprocedural voice therapy in spasmodic dysphonia remains unclear at this time.

Essential voice tremor may manifest in up to 10–25% of patients with essential tremor [80, 86]. This is typically treated with botulinum toxin injections or alternatively medications, with voice therapy playing less of a central role [87]. When employed, voice therapy focuses on behavioral modification to decrease listener perception of tremor [88, 89]. To the authors' knowledge, no studies to date have evaluated the effect of including voice therapy treatment perioperatively in this patient group.

Parkinson disease-related voice disorders also may include a variety of treatments. The gold standard of voice therapy for these patients is Lee Silverman Voice Treatment, a direct voice therapy focusing on recognizing the increased vocal effort needed to produce adequate speaking volume [32, 80].

15.9 Timing

Perioperative voice therapy may be divided into the preoperative and postoperative time periods. Voice therapy in both time periods should facilitate setting patient expectations and facilitating the optimization of the postoperative voice.

15.9.1 Preoperative Therapy

Preoperative voice therapy may serve several functions. As described in Tang and Thibeault 2017 for BVFLs, it may address various aspects of postoperative care important to optimizing the result following procedural intervention, including: "general vocal hygiene, immediate postoperative voice care, and recovery expectations" [90]. This study found that in those who received even one preoperative therapy session had statistically significant improvement in their Vocal Handicap Index scores, which those who were only given postoperative voice therapy did not. The authors postulate that this may be analogous to pre- and postoperative therapy benefits in orthopedics, but also theorize that setting expectations with patients regarding voicing following phonosurgery increases patients' perceived benefit [90].

Sahin et al. 2018 compared outcomes in 3 groups of patients with vocal fold polyps: (1) those who were treated with 10, 40-45 min voice therapy sessions, (2) those who were treated with surgical excision alone, and (3) those who received voice therapy followed by surgical intervention. Group 3 had the greatest treatment success of the three groups, suggesting that preoperative therapy is a useful adjunct [48].

Apart from data generated from patients with BVFLs, there has been limited investigation of the role of preprocedural voice therapy. In Heuer et al. 1997, many patients with vocal fold paresis who were treated with an average of 3 voice therapy sessions preoperatively did not subsequently require procedural intervention [67]. Gartner-Schmidt and Rosen reported in their 2011 study of vocal fold atrophy treatment that patients treated with voice therapy and subsequent surgery had lower rates of treatment success (17%) compared with those receiving either intervention alone (surgery = 56%, voice therapy = 36%). However, it should be noted that treatment success was based on an improvement on Voice Handicap Index of greater than 5 points, and when asked whether they believed it had helped them, 81% of patients who had been treated with voice therapy responded "Yes" [78]. Additionally, sample sizes in this study were low, and further investigation is warranted to determine the utility of preprocedural voice therapy in this population.

15.9.2 Postoperative Voice Rest

A comprehensive review of voice rest is beyond the scope of this chapter, but it is of note that there are currently no standard recommendations for voice rest following phonosurgery. Clinicians vary significantly in the type (absolute vs. relative) and duration of voice rest they recommend. A 2003 study of American otolaryngologists detailed that 51.4% favored absolute voice rest, 62.3% favored relative voice rest, and 15.1% of physicians advocated for neither type of voice rest. In those physicians recommending absolute or relative voice rest, the average length of intervention was 7 days [91]. A more recent survey of British otolaryngologists revealed that in benign vocal fold lesions, relative voice rest was recommended 40.9–46.3% of the time, while absolute voice rest was advised 11.7–25.8% of the time and no voice rest was advised 8.6–31.5% of the time. The most commonly advised duration of voice rest was 1–2 days, however many physicians advocated for 7 or more days [92].

Apart from differences in clinician preference, patients find it difficult to comply with absolute, rather than relative, voice rest [25, 93]. This introduces difficulty in comparing the two options in a research setting, and may lead to greater rates of persistent postoperative dysphonia in patients advised to attempt extended courses of absolute voice rest [25, 94].

Randomized clinical trials evaluating optimal duration of voice rest are limited. One such study of 31 patients with benign vocal fold lesions indicated that a 3-day period of absolute voice rest resulted in improved mucosal function as measured by normalized mucosal wave amplitude 6 months following phonosurgery when compared with 7 days of rest. However, no other acoustic or patient-reported outcome measure demonstrated a statistically significant difference in voice quality between the two groups [95].

15.9.3 Other Postoperative Therapy

Apart from voice rest in the immediate postoperative period, ongoing rehabilitative voice therapy may be used to attempt to improve postoperative voice quality [37, 49–52, 79] or decrease recurrence of laryngeal pathology [38]. Several authors have described postoperative voice therapy in those with BVFLs. In patients with vocal fold polyp treated with phonomicrosurgery, You et al. report that in patients provided with postoperative education about proper voice use as well as relaxation, breathing, vocal function, and other direct exercises, there was an improvement in self-rated voice quality relative to those who did not receive postoperative voice therapy [52]. Ju similarly found in patients with vocal fold polyps, two 30-minute sessions of voice therapy in the fourth week following phonomicrosurgery, which consisted of both indirect interventions and direct therapies such as vocal resonance exercises, could improve subjective voice outcomes [51]. As described in Sect. 15.5, Petrovic-Lazic et al. and Lin et al. also found that postoperative voice therapy, involving both indirect and direct therapy components, improved subjective and objective voice outcomes following phonomicrosurgery for vocal fold polyp [49, 50].

Not all BVFLs have evidence to support the efficacy of postoperative voice therapy. As detailed in Sect. 15.5, a study by Tibbetts et al. in patients with vocal fold cysts failed to find significant benefit of postoperative voice therapy. The voice therapy protocol used in this study was not specified, however, and the majority of the cysts in this patient population were mucus retention cysts rather than epidermal inclusion cysts. The authors theorized these cysts to be less responsive to voice therapy than other histologic subtypes as they are not thought to be closely related to phonotrauma [53].

Apart from BVFLs, there is minimal literature describing the use of postoperative voice therapy in other conditions. In two cases of vocal fold bowing (described in Sect. 15.7), 3 months of vocal function exercises were used with the effect of improving subjective and objective voice measures [79]. There is mixed evidence for the use of postprocedural voice therapy in patients with spasmodic dysphonia (Sect. 15.8). Murry and Woodson found benefit in 17 patients who returned following vocal fold injection for direct interventions centered around decreasing vocal effort and increasing continuous airflow during phonation [83]. In contrast, Silverman et al. did not replicate this result in 10 patients treated with voice therapy centered around "minimization of voice hyperfunction through voice education, relaxation, laryngeal massage" [85].

15.10 Frequency and Duration

Where described, published data discussing the length of voice therapy in the perioperative period ranges significantly, as no universal standard exists. Preoperative voice therapy may be limited to a single session, in many cases focused on preoperative counseling and vocal hygiene [51, 90, 95, 96]. Alternatively, it may include multiple voice therapy appointments, some spanning one to several months and using a combination of indirect and direct techniques [47, 48, 52, 96–98]. Barillari et al. describe a standard set of 8, 30-min preoperative sessions twice weekly preoperatively in their patient population, while Sahin et al. assigned patients to 10, 40–45-min twice weekly appointments prior to phonosurgery [47, 48]. Few other studies fully describe frequency and duration of preoperative therapy.

Rehabilitative postoperative voice therapy, following periods of voice rest, is similarly variable. In a 2000 article, Rosen et al. describe a range of 6–16 weeks of postoperative voice therapy, with 6–13 sessions contained within that timeframe [96]. Kaneko et al. limited postoperative therapy to 6 weeks, citing decreased patient compliance beyond this timeframe [95]. When studying patients status-post surgical treatment of vocal fold polyp, Kunduk et al. note only two sessions of voice therapy, 1 and 3 months postoperatively [41]. In a retrospective review of 55 patients who had received voice therapy following vocal polyp excision, Ju et al. report patients received 2, 30-min sessions in the fourth week following their procedure [51]. Much sooner after polyp removal, Petrovic-Lazic et al. reported three weekly sessions of voice therapy, beginning 10 days following phonomicrosurgery and continuing for 4 weeks [49]. More recently, in 2017 Barillari et al. describe 8, 30-minute sessions twice weekly 15 days following surgery, and You et al. report one 60–90-min session every 2 weeks for 3 months after phonosurgery, with emphasis on individual practice of vocal exercises at home [47, 52].

This wide range of reported voice therapy frequency and duration perioperatively is reflective of voice therapy as a primary treatment. In a 2017 review of voice therapy used to treat organic and functional voice disorders, patients received therapy on average 1–2 times weekly for 40.74 min each session. They had an average of 10.5 total sessions, resulting in 8.73 h of average total therapy. However, this ranged from 3 to 18 total hours [15]. Previous studies noted similar variability, including voice improvement as measured by pitch modification from only one voice therapy session [13, 99].

Optimal scheduling of perioperative voice therapy is an area of opportunity for future research, as current reported protocols in the literature are disparate and largely without strong evidence or explicit reasoning for their frequency or duration. Currently, as with other aspects of perioperative therapy, treatment course would best be established individually based on the patient's needs, access to care and recommendations from their SLP.

15.11 Factors Predictive of Successful Voice Therapy

A variety of factors, both modifiable and not, may impact the extent of benefit patients receive from voice therapy. Adherence to voice therapy, for both direct and indirect interventions, is challenging for some patients and decreased compliance with therapy may limit postoperative voice recovery [25, 100]. In addition to adherence, the patient's ability to complete the type of voice therapy an SLP uses may impact their eventual voice outcome. Carding et al. suggest that indirect therapies in particular are more effective for patients that can independently identify voice stressors, accept that these stressors may contribute to dysphonia, and respond positively to the idea of modifying these stressors [7].

In studies describing voice therapy for BVFLs, there are several patient factors that correlate with a greater likelihood of treatment success. In patients with vocal fold polyps, those with small [22, 42, 43, 101, 102], sessile [43], and translucent, non-hemorrhagic [44, 101] lesions are more likely to respond to voice therapy. Women with vocal fold polyps may be more likely to improve compared to men [42, 43], as well as patients with mild to moderate (rather than severe) occupational voice demands and those who have had a shorter duration of dysphonia [22, 42, 102]. There is mixed evidence as to whether smoking tobacco portends a poor response to voice therapy in those with vocal fold polyp [22].

Early referral to voice therapy may also be of importance in terms of increasing likelihood of a response, and by doing so improving quality of life, in patients with vocal fold paralysis [59, 62, 65]. However, there is also literature to suggest that patients may still experience improved voice impairment with delayed treatment, and there is currently no conclusive time course for voice therapy in this population [61, 63]. Of note, Heuer et al. suggest that in patients with vocal fold paralysis after unilateral recurrent laryngeal nerve injury, those with an inability to complete glottal closure are unlikely to respond to voice therapy alone [67].

In patients with spasmodic dysphonia, it has been suggested that those with persistent extrinsic muscular compensation following botulinum toxin injection of the vocal fold may benefit most from postprocedural voice therapy, as it is possible to resolve this with direct interventions [83].

Key Learning Points:

- SLPs should be involved early and longitudinally in the patient's treatment course, following endoscopic examination and determination of the etiology of dysphonia.
- Both indirect and direct voice therapy methods have been shown to benefit patients and may be used perioperatively: the proportion of each intervention should be assigned on an individualized basis. Perioperative therapy may include both education regarding voice hygiene and expected postoperative change, as well as direct therapies to optimize voicing following procedural intervention.
- Many patients undergoing procedural intervention to the vocal folds are appropriate for the use of voice therapy, either as a primary treatment prior to surgery or as an adjunct, as this has been shown to improve outcomes in a variety of conditions.
- Both pre- and postoperative voice therapy may benefit voice outcomes, and it is the authors' recommendation that both be offered to patients undergoing laryngeal procedures.
- Given the current lack of conclusive evidence regarding standardization of perioperative voice therapy content, timing, frequency and duration, patients' precise treatment courses should be established individually with their SLP.
- Patient commitment and adherence to voice therapy is pivotal in its success.
- In those with vocal fold polyps, voice therapy is more likely to be successful with lesions that are small, sessile and non-hemorrhagic. Additional modifying factors may include sex, occupational voice demands, onset of dysphonia, and smoking status.
- Early involvement of speech-language pathology is important in all etiologies of dysphonia being considered for surgical intervention but may be of particular importance in vocal fold paralysis due to delays potentially impacting voice therapy response.

References

1. Stachler RJ, Francis DO, Schwartz SR, Damask CC, Digoy GP, Krouse HJ, et al. Clinical practice guideline: hoarseness (Dysphonia) (Update). Otolaryngol Head Neck Surg. 2018;158(1 suppl):S1-S42.
2. Woo P, Colton R, Casper J, Brewer D. Diagnostic value of stroboscopic examination in hoarse patients. J Voice; 1991. p. 231–238.
3. Bergeron M, Kelchner L, Weinrich B, Brehm SB, Zacharias S, Myer C, et al. Influence of preoperative voice assessment on treatment plan prior to airway surgery. Laryngoscope. 2018;128(12):2858–63.
4. Teppo H, Alho OP. Relative importance of diagnostic delays in different head and neck cancers. Clin Otolaryngol. 2008;33(4):325–30.
5. Teppo H, Alho OP. Comorbidity and diagnostic delay in cancer of the larynx, tongue and pharynx. Oral Oncol. 2009;45(8):692–5.
6. Van Stan JH, Roy N, Awan S, Stemple J, Hillman RE. A taxonomy of voice therapy. Am J Speech Lang Pathol. 2015;24(2):101–25.
7. Carding PN, Horsley IA, Docherty GJ. A study of the effectiveness of voice therapy in the treatment of 45 patients with nonorganic dysphonia. J Voice. 1999;13(1):72–104.
8. Thomas L. Voice therapy: does science support the art? In: Stemple J, editor.: Communicative disorders review; 2007. p. 49–77.
9. Roy N, Gray SD, Simon M, Dove H, Corbin-Lewis K, Stemple JC. An evaluation of the effects of two treatment approaches for teachers with voice disorders: a prospective randomized clinical trial. J Speech Lang Hear Res. 2001;44(2):286–96.
10. Ruotsalainen J, Sellman J, Lehto L, Verbeek J. Systematic review of the treatment of functional dysphonia and prevention of voice disorders. Otolaryngol Head Neck Surg. 2008;138(5):557–65.
11. MacKenzie K, Millar A, Wilson JA, Sellars C, Deary IJ. Is voice therapy an effective treatment for dysphonia? A randomised controlled trial. BMJ. 2001;323(7314):658–61.
12. Gillivan-Murphy P, Drinnan MJ, O'Dwyer TP, Ridha H, Carding P. The effectiveness of a voice treatment

approach for teachers with self-reported voice problems. J Voice. 2006;20(3):423–31.
13. Speyer R. Effects of voice therapy: a systematic review. J Voice. 2008;22(5):565–80.
14. Roy N, Weinrich B, Gray SD, Tanner K, Toledo SW, Dove H, et al. Voice amplification versus vocal hygiene instruction for teachers with voice disorders: a treatment outcomes study. J Speech Lang Hear Res. 2002;45(4):625–38.
15. Desjardins M, Halstead L, Cooke M, Bonilha HS. A systematic review of voice therapy: what "Effectiveness" really implies. J Voice. 2017;31(3):392.e13-.e32.
16. Behrman A, Rutledge J, Hembree A, Sheridan S. Vocal hygiene education, voice production therapy, and the role of patient adherence: a treatment effectiveness study in women with phonotrauma. J Speech Lang Hear Res. 2008;51(2):350–66.
17. Rodríguez-Parra MJ, Adrián JA, Casado JC. Comparing voice-therapy and vocal-hygiene treatments in dysphonia using a limited multidimensional evaluation protocol. J Commun Disord. 2011;44(6):615–30.
18. Watts CR, Hamilton A, Toles L, Childs L, Mau T. A randomized controlled trial of stretch-and-flow voice therapy for muscle tension dysphonia. Laryngoscope. 2015;125(6):1420–5.
19. Ziegler A, Dastolfo C, Hersan R, Rosen CA, Gartner-Schmidt J. Perceptions of voice therapy from patients diagnosed with primary muscle tension dysphonia and benign mid-membranous vocal fold lesions. J Voice. 2014;28(6):742–52.
20. Gartner-Schmidt JL, Roth DF, Zullo TG, Rosen CA. Quantifying component parts of indirect and direct voice therapy related to different voice disorders. J Voice. 2013;27(2):210–6.
21. Chan RW. Does the voice improve with vocal hygiene education? A study of some instrumental voice measures in a group of kindergarten teachers. J Voice. 1994;8(3):279–91.
22. Yun YS, Kim MB, Son YI. The effect of vocal hygiene education for patients with vocal polyp. Otolaryngol Head Neck Surg. 2007;137(4):569–75.
23. Pasa G, Oates J, Dacakis G. The relative effectiveness of vocal hygiene training and vocal function exercises in preventing voice disorders in primary school teachers. Logoped Phoniatr Vocol. 2007;32(3):128–40.
24. Koufman JA, Blalock PD. Classification and approach to patients with functional voice disorders. Ann Otol Rhinol Laryngol. 1982;91(4 Pt 1):372–7.
25. Koufman JA, Blalock PD. Is voice rest never indicated? J Voice. 1989;3:87–91.
26. Dejonckere PH, Bradley P, Clemente P, Cornut G, Crevier-Buchman L, Friedrich G, et al. A basic protocol for functional assessment of voice pathology, especially for investigating the efficacy of (phonosurgical) treatments and evaluating new assessment techniques. Guideline elaborated by the committee on Phoniatrics of the European laryngological society (ELS). Eur Arch Otorhinolaryngol. 2001;258(2):77–82.
27. Lopes LW, da Silva JD, Simões LB, Evangelista DDS, Silva POC, Almeida AA, et al. Relationship between acoustic measurements and self-evaluation in patients with voice disorders. J Voice. 2017;31(1):119.e1-.e10.
28. Schindler A, Mozzanica F, Vedrody M, Maruzzi P, Ottaviani F. Correlation between the voice handicap index and voice measurements in four groups of patients with dysphonia. Otolaryngol Head Neck Surg. 2009;141(6):762–9.
29. Kiagiadaki DE, Chimona TS, Chlouverakis GI, Stylianou Y, Proimos EK, Papadakis CE, et al. Evaluating the outcome of phonosurgery: comparing the role of VHI and VoiSS questionnaires in the Greek language. J Voice. 2012;26(3):372–7.
30. Rosen CA, Gartner-Schmidt J, Hathaway B, Simpson CB, Postma GN, Courey M, et al. A nomenclature paradigm for benign midmembranous vocal fold lesions. Laryngoscope. 2012;122(6):1335–41.
31. Schindler A, Mozzanica F, Ginocchio D, Maruzzi P, Atac M, Ottaviani F. Vocal improvement after voice therapy in the treatment of benign vocal fold lesions. Acta Otorhinolaryngol Ital. 2012;32(5): 304–8.
32. Carding P, Bos-Clark M, Fu S, Gillivan-Murphy P, Jones SM, Walton C. Evaluating the efficacy of voice therapy for functional, organic and neurological voice disorders. Clin Otolaryngol. 2017;42(2):201–17.
33. Kraimer KL, Husain I. Updated medical and surgical treatment for common benign laryngeal lesions. Otolaryngol Clin N Am. 2019;52(4):745–57.
34. Akbulut S, Gartner-Schmidt JL, Gillespie AI, Young VN, Smith LJ, Rosen CA. Voice outcomes following treatment of benign midmembranous vocal fold lesions using a nomenclature paradigm. Laryngoscope. 2016;126(2):415–20.
35. Johns MM, Garrett CG, Hwang J, Ossoff RH, Courey MS. Quality-of-life outcomes following laryngeal endoscopic surgery for non-neoplastic vocal fold lesions. Ann Otol Rhinol Laryngol. 2004;113(8):597–601.
36. Mansuri B, Tohidast SA, Soltaninejad N, Kamali M, Ghelichi L, Azimi H. Nonmedical treatments of vocal fold nodules: a systematic review. J Voice. 2018;32(5):609–20.
37. Murry T, Woodson G. A comparison of three methods for the management of vocal fold nodules. J Voice. 1992. p. 271–276.
38. Béquignon E, Bach C, Fugain C, Guilleré L, Blumen M, Chabolle F, et al. Long-term results of surgical treatment of vocal fold nodules. Laryngoscope. 2013;123(8):1926–30.
39. Sulica L, Behrman A. Management of benign vocal fold lesions: a survey of current opinion and practice. Ann Otol Rhinol Laryngol. 2003;112(10):827–33.

40. White A. Management of benign vocal fold lesions: current perspectives on the role for voice therapy. Curr Opin Otolaryngol Head Neck Surg. 2019;27(3):185–90.
41. Kunduk M, Dölinger M, McWhorter AJ, Svec JG, Lohscheller J. Vocal fold vibratory behavior changes following surgical treatment of polyps investigated with high-speed videoendoscopy and phonovibrography. Ann Otol Rhinol Laryngol. 2012;121(6):355–63.
42. Nakagawa H, Miyamoto M, Kusuyama T, Mori Y, Fukuda H. Resolution of vocal fold polyps with conservative treatment. J Voice. 2012;26(3):e107–10.
43. Lee YS, Lee DH, Jeong GE, Kim JW, Roh JL, Choi SH, et al. Treatment efficacy of voice therapy for vocal fold polyps and factors predictive of its efficacy. J Voice. 2017;31(1):120.e9-.e13.
44. Cohen SM, Garrett CG. Utility of voice therapy in the management of vocal fold polyps and cysts. Otolaryngol Head Neck Surg. 2007;136(5):742–6.
45. Zhuge P, You H, Wang H, Zhang Y, Du H. An analysis of the effects of voice therapy on patients with early vocal fold polyps. J Voice. 2016;30(6):698–704.
46. Wang H, Zhuge P, You H, Zhang Y, Zhang Z. Comparison of the efficacy of vocal training and vocal microsurgery in patients with early vocal fold polyp. Braz J Otorhinolaryngol. 2019;85(6):678–84.
47. Barillari MR, Volpe U, Mirra G, Giugliano F, Barillari U. Surgery or rehabilitation: a randomized clinical trial comparing the treatment of vocal fold polyps via phonosurgery and traditional voice therapy with "Voice Therapy Expulsion" training. J Voice. 2017;31(3):379.e13-.e20.
48. Sahin M, Gode S, Dogan M, Kirazli T, Ogut F. Effect of voice therapy on vocal fold polyp treatment. Eur Arch Otorhinolaryngol. 2018;275(6):1533–40.
49. Petrovic-Lazic M, Jovanovic N, Kulic M, Babac S, Jurisic V. Acoustic and perceptual characteristics of the voice in patients with vocal polyps after surgery and voice therapy. J Voice. 2015;29(2):241–6.
50. Lin L, Sun N, Yang Q, Zhang Y, Shen J, Shi L, et al. Effect of voice training in the voice rehabilitation of patients with vocal cord polyps after surgery. Exp Ther Med. 2014;7(4):877–80.
51. Ju YH, Jung KY, Kwon SY, Woo JS, Cho JG, Park MW, et al. Effect of voice therapy after phonomicrosurgery for vocal polyps: a prospective, historically controlled, clinical study. J Laryngol Otol. 2013;127(11):1134–8.
52. You Ha, Zhuge P, Wang H, **Zhang Y**, Du H. Clinical observation of the effect of voice training on patients with vocal cord polyps after phonomicrosurgery. Biomed Res; 2017. p. 3874–3879.
53. Tibbetts KM, Dominguez LM, Simpson CB. Impact of perioperative voice therapy on outcomes in the surgical Management of Vocal Fold Cysts. J Voice. 2018;32(3):347–51.
54. Leonard R, Kendall K. Effects of voice therapy on vocal process granuloma: a phonoscopic approach. Am J Otolaryngol. 2005;26(2):101–7.
55. Ylitalo R, Hammarberg B. Voice characteristics, effects of voice therapy, and long-term follow-up of contact granuloma patients. J Voice. 2000;14(4):557–66.
56. White AC, Carding P. Pre- and postoperative voice therapy for benign vocal fold lesions: factors influencing a complex intervention. J Voice. 2020;
57. Pedersen M, McGlashan J. Surgical versus non-surgical interventions for vocal cord nodules. Cochrane Database Syst Rev. 2012;6:CD001934.
58. Kelchner LN, Stemple JC, Gerdeman E, Le Borgne W, Adam S. Etiology, pathophysiology, treatment choices, and voice results for unilateral adductor vocal fold paralysis: a 3-year retrospective. J Voice. 1999;13(4):592–601.
59. D'Alatri L, Galla S, Rigante M, Antonelli O, Buldrini S, Marchese MR. Role of early voice therapy in patients affected by unilateral vocal fold paralysis. J Laryngol Otol. 2008;122(9):936–41.
60. Schindler A, Bottero A, Capaccio P, Ginocchio D, Adorni F, Ottaviani F. Vocal improvement after voice therapy in unilateral vocal fold paralysis. J Voice. 2008;22(1):113–8.
61. Cantarella G, Viglione S, Forti S, Pignataro L. Voice therapy for laryngeal hemiplegia: the role of timing of initiation of therapy. J Rehabil Med. 2010;42(5):442–6.
62. El-Banna M, Youssef G. Early voice therapy in patients with unilateral vocal fold paralysis. Folia Phoniatr Logop. 2014;66(6):237–43.
63. Busto-Crespo O, Uzcanga-Lacabe M, Abad-Marco A, Berasategui I, García L, Maraví E, et al. Longitudinal Voice Outcomes After Voice Therapy in Unilateral Vocal Fold Paralysis. J Voice. 2016;30(6):767.e9-.e15.
64. Khidr A. Effects of the "Smith Accent Technique" of voice therapy on the laryngeal functions and voice quality of patients with unilateral vocal fold paralysis. Int Congr Ser 2003. p. 1235–1241.
65. Mattioli F, Menichetti M, Bergamini G, Molteni G, Alberici MP, Luppi MP, et al. Results of early versus intermediate or delayed voice therapy in patients with unilateral vocal fold paralysis: our experience in 171 patients. J Voice. 2015;29(4):455–8.
66. Walton C, Conway E, Blackshaw H, Carding P. Unilateral vocal fold paralysis: a systematic review of speech-language pathology management. J Voice. 2017;31(4):509.e7-.e22.
67. Heuer RJ, Sataloff RT, Emerich K, Rulnick R, Baroody M, Spiegel JR, et al. Unilateral recurrent laryngeal nerve paralysis: the importance of "preoperative" voice therapy. J Voice. 1997;11(1):88–94.
68. Kendall K. Presbyphonia: a review. Curr Opin Otolaryngol Head Neck Surg. 2007;15(3):137–40.
69. Sachs AM, Bielamowicz SA, Stager SV. Treatment effectiveness for aging changes in the larynx. Laryngoscope. 2017;127(11):2572–7.
70. Ziegler A, Verdolini Abbott K, Johns M, Klein A, Hapner ER. Preliminary data on two voice therapy

interventions in the treatment of presbyphonia. Laryngoscope. 2014;124(8):1869–76.
71. Lu FL, Presley S, Lammers B. Efficacy of intensive phonatory-respiratory treatment (LSVT) for presbyphonia: two case reports. J Voice. 2013;27(6):786.e11–23.
72. Tay EY, Phyland DJ, Oates J. The effect of vocal function exercises on the voices of aging community choral singers. J Voice. 2012;26(5):672.e19–27.
73. Godoy J, Silverio K, Brasolotto A. Effectiveness of vocal therapy for the elderly when applying conventional and intensive approaches: a randomized clinical trial. J Voice. 2019;33(5):809.e19-.e26.
74. Guzman M, Saldivar P, Pérez R, Muñoz D. Aerodynamic, Electroglottographic, and acoustic outcomes after tube phonation in water in elderly subjects. Folia Phoniatr Logop. 2018;70(3–4):149–55.
75. Lagorio LA, Carnaby-Mann GD, Crary MA. Treatment of vocal fold bowing using neuromuscular electrical stimulation. Arch Otolaryngol Head Neck Surg. 2010;136(4):398–403.
76. Sauder C, Roy N, Tanner K, Houtz DR, Smith ME. Vocal function exercises for presbylaryngis: a multidimensional assessment of treatment outcomes. Ann Otol Rhinol Laryngol. 2010;119(7):460–7.
77. Berg EE, Hapner E, Klein A, Johns MM. Voice therapy improves quality of life in age-related dysphonia: a case-control study. J Voice. 2008;22(1):70–4.
78. Gartner-Schmidt J, Rosen C. Treatment success for age-related vocal fold atrophy. Laryngoscope. 2011;121(3):585–9.
79. Tanner K, Sauder C, Thibeault SL, Dromey C, Smith ME. Vocal fold bowing in elderly male monozygotic twins: a case study. J Voice. 2010;24(4):470–6.
80. Snow G, Guardiani E. Movement disorders and voice. Otolaryngol Clin N Am. 2019;52(4):759–67.
81. Sulica L. Contemporary management of spasmodic dysphonia. Curr Opin Otolaryngol Head Neck Surg. 2004;12(6):543–8.
82. Bloch CS, Hirano M, Gould WJ. Symptom improvement of spastic dysphonia in response to phonatory tasks. Ann Otol Rhinol Laryngol. 1985;94(1 Pt 1):51–4.
83. Murry T, Woodson GE. Combined-modality treatment of adductor spasmodic dysphonia with botulinum toxin and voice therapy. J Voice. 1995;9(4):460–5.
84. Paniello RC, Edgar JD, Perlmutter JS. Vocal exercise versus voice rest following botulinum toxin injections: a randomized crossover trial. Ann Otol Rhinol Laryngol. 2009;118(11):759–63.
85. Silverman EP, Garvan C, Shrivastav R, Sapienza CM. Combined modality treatment of adductor spasmodic dysphonia. J Voice. 2012;26(1):77–86.
86. Patel A, Frucht SJ. Isolated vocal tremor as a focal phenotype of essential tremor: a retrospective case review. J Clin Mov Disord. 2015;2:4.
87. Sulica L, Louis ED. Clinical characteristics of essential voice tremor: a study of 34 cases. Laryngoscope. 2010;120(3):516–28.
88. Barkmeier-Kraemer J. Updates on vocal tremor and its management. Perspectives on Voice and Voice Disorders. 2012;22(3):97–103.
89. Barkmeier-Kraemer J, Lato A, Wiley K. Development of a speech treatment program for a client with essential vocal tremor. Semin Speech Lang. 2011;32(1):43–57.
90. Tang SS, Thibeault SL. Timing of voice therapy: a primary investigation of voice outcomes for surgical benign vocal fold lesion patients. J Voice. 2017;31(1):129.e1-.e7.
91. Behrman A, Sulica L. Voice rest after microlaryngoscopy: current opinion and practice. Laryngoscope. 2003;113(12):2182–6.
92. Coombs AC, Carswell AJ, Tierney PA. Voice rest after vocal fold surgery: current practice and evidence. J Laryngol Otol. 2013;127(8):773–9.
93. Whitling S, Lyberg-Åhlander V, Rydell R. Absolute or relative voice rest after phonosurgery: a blind randomized prospective clinical trial. Logoped Phoniatr Vocol. 2018;43(4):143–54.
94. Ishikawa K, Thibeault S. Voice rest versus exercise: a review of the literature. J Voice. 2010;24(4):379–87.
95. Kaneko M, Shiromoto O, Fujiu-Kurachi M, Kishimoto Y, Tateya I, Hirano S. Optimal duration for voice rest after vocal fold surgery: randomized controlled clinical study. J Voice. 2017;31(1):97–103.
96. Rosen CA, Murry T, Zinn A, Zullo T, Sonbolian M. Voice handicap index change following treatment of voice disorders. J Voice. 2000;14(4):619–23.
97. do Amaral Catani GS, Hamerschmidt R, Moreira AT, Timi JR, Wiemes GR, Ido J, et al. Subjective and objective analyses of voice improvement after Phonosurgery in professional voice users. Med Probl Perform Art. 2016;31(1):18–24.
98. Estes C, Sulica L. Vocal fold pseudocyst: results of 46 cases undergoing a uniform treatment algorithm. Laryngoscope. 2014;124(5):1180–6.
99. Roy N, Hendarto H. Revisiting the pitch controversy: changes in speaking fundamental frequency (SFF) after management of functional dysphonia. J Voice. 2005;19(4):582–91.
100. Portone C, Johns MM, Hapner ER. A review of patient adherence to the recommendation for voice therapy. J Voice. 2008;22(2):192–6.
101. Cho KJ, Nam IC, Hwang YS, Shim MR, Park JO, Cho JH, et al. Analysis of factors influencing voice quality and therapeutic approaches in vocal polyp patients. Eur Arch Otorhinolaryngol. 2011;268(9):1321–7.
102. Klein AM, Lehmann M, Hapner ER, Johns MM. Spontaneous resolution of hemorrhagic polyps of the true vocal fold. J Voice. 2009;23(1):132–5.

Part V

Special Considerations in Various Vocal Fold Injections

Botulinum Toxin Injection for Laryngeal Disorders

16

Jae-Yol Lim

Abstract

Laryngeal botulinum toxin injection is an essential treatment for spasmodic dysphonia (SD) and other laryngeal disorders, including essential laryngeal voice tremor, muscle tension dysphonia, vocal fold granuloma, and chronic cough. Botulinum neurotoxin type A (BoNTA) is the most commonly used formulation for treating patients diagnosed with SD. Injecting BoNTA into the adductor thyroarytenoid or abductor posterior cricoarytenoid muscles inhibits acetylcholine release at the neuromuscular junction and reduces muscular hyperactivity by chemical denervation. A randomized, double-blind, sham-controlled trial reported BoNTA injection as an effective treatment for patients with SD, and numerous studies have subsequently reported its efficacy and safety in the treatment of SD over the past 30 years. Guidelines for administering BoNTA injections are not well standardized and are usually individualized based on the patient's vocal demands, treatment responses, and side effects. However, clinical strategies for administering BoNTA injections do not significantly differ among laryngologists. In this chapter, general principles, treatment protocols, and techniques of administering laryngeal BoNTA injection for the treatment of adductor or abductor SD are discussed. In addition, other applications of laryngeal BoNTA injection are also addressed.

Keywords

Vocal fold injection · Botulinum toxin
Spasmodic dysphonia · Laryngeal disorders

16.1 Treatment of Adductor Spasmodic Dysphonia

Spasmodic dysphonia (SD) is a rare voice disorder caused by laryngeal dystonia that is characterized by involuntary voice breaks and increased vocal efforts during speech but not initially during innate vocalization such as crying, laughing, shouting, whispering, singing, or yawning. Adductor SD features spasmodic hyperadduction of the vocal folds, leading to intermittent disruption of phonation with strained and strangulated voice quality. Abductor SD is less common, and patients present with hyperabduction of the vocal folds, leading to prolonged voiceless consonants before vowel phonation [1]. A three-tiered approach, including a questionnaire, speech assessment, and nasolaryngoscopy, is generally recommended for the diagnosis of SD [2]. The distinguishing sign of SD is the occurrence of

J.-Y. Lim (✉)
Department of Otorhinolaryngology, Gangnam Severance Hospital, Yonsei University College of Medicine, Seoul, Republic of Korea
e-mail: jylimmd@yuhs.ac

© Springer Nature Singapore Pte Ltd. 2021
B.-J. Lee et al. (eds.), *Vocal Fold Injection*, https://doi.org/10.1007/978-981-16-3303-4_16

voice breaks during spontaneous speech, which can be documented using acoustic and aerodynamic assessments [3]. Task specificity is another major diagnostic characteristic of SD, and the severity of dysphonia for patients is significantly greater during connected speech than during sustained vowel phonation [4]. In contrast, this phenomenon is not a characteristic of patients with muscle tension dysphonia [4]. Despite recent advances in identifying possible risk factors and the pathogenesis of SD, accurate diagnosis is delayed because of the lack of objective diagnostic criteria and variations in voice manifestations with the heterogeneity of patient populations.

16.1.1 General Principles of BoNTA Injection for Adductor SD

Botulinum neurotoxin type A (BoNTA, Botox; Allergan, Inc., Irvine, CA, USA) has been the first-line treatment for patients diagnosed with adductor SD [5]. Injecting BoNTA into the adductor thyroarytenoid (TA) muscle leads to the inhibition of acetylcholine release at the neuromuscular junction and reduced muscular hyperactivity by chemical denervation [6]. The goal of therapy is to alleviate voice breaks and reduce vocal efforts without causing significant breathiness of the voice. Although the BoNTA injection guidelines are not well standardized and are usually individualized based on patients' vocal demands, treatment responses, and side effects, clinical practices of administering BoNTA injections do not differ significantly among laryngologists [7]. For the treatment of adductor SD, the office-based trans-cervical (trans-cricothyroid) approach, electromyography (EMG)-guided injection, and bilateral injection of BoNTA are preferentially used [8]. The key to successful treatment management is the consistent placement of the injection and individual dose titration. BoNTA can also be injected trans-orally or using the trans-thyrohyoid approach with indirect or flexible laryngoscopic guidance [9]. Moreover, experienced physicians can achieve accurate placement and comparable results using percutaneous injection without EMG guidance [10].

16.1.2 Treatment Protocols of BoNTA Injection for Adductor SD

Initial administration of low-dose BoNTA injection is feasible even in patients with severe dysphonia. Blitzer et al. [11] recommended several individualized injection strategies depending on the patient's response, with an average dose of 0.9 IU/0.1 mL per vocal fold for bilateral injections and 1.5 IU/0.1 mL for unilateral injections [11]. A recent study by Rosow et al. [12] showed that a relatively low initial BoNTA dose could be used in all patients with adductor SD [12]. Although bilateral BoNTA injections are commonly used, unilateral BoNTA injections using adequate dosing and follow-up protocols have also been advocated as an excellent option to reduce side effects with comparable efficacy to bilateral BoNTA injections [13]. Although the efficacy and safety of unilateral injections have been reported, there are some disagreements concerning its protocols. Unilateral injections can be administered on the same side until BoNTA becomes ineffective or, alternatingly, to each vocal fold at every visit [14]. The unilateral injection strategy commonly involves administering 1–3 units/side with a median of 1.5 IU/side [15]. Nevertheless, most laryngologists prefer to start with bilateral injections at an initial dose of 1.25 units/side ranging from 0.25 to 5 units [7]. The optimal dose is determined after a short trial period, and then unilateral or bilateral BoNTA injections are subsequently repeated according to the patient's response (Fig. 16.1).

Periodic BoNTA injections have been considered the gold standard for the treatment of adductor SD. Subsequent doses are then determined according to the patient's age, sex, past history, and treatment response, such as duration of improved phonation after BoNTA injection and tolerance to post-injection side effects [16]. BoNTA injection induces thyroarytenoid (TA) muscle weakness and ameliorates speech interruption and the strained or strangled voice quality associated with adductor SD. However, its limitations include the need for repeated injections, short-term swallowing and voice problems after injection, and the unpredictable relationship

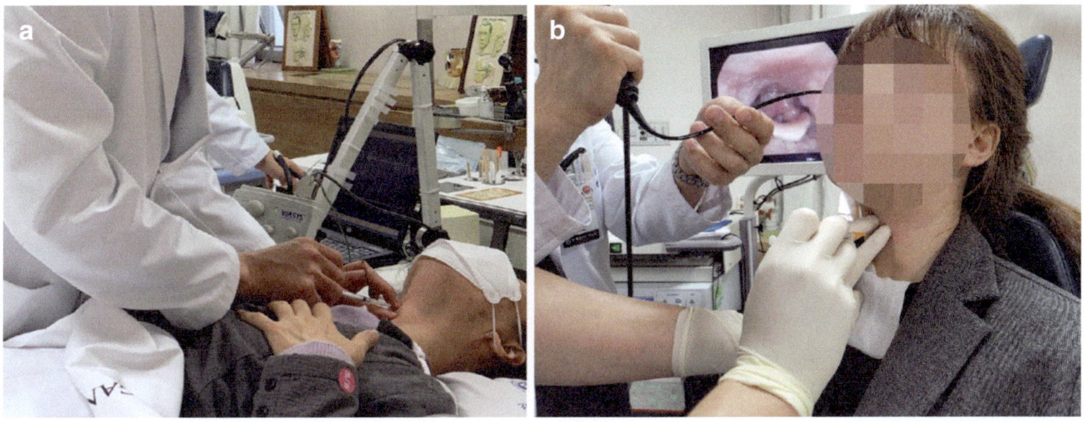

Fig. 16.1 Botulinum neurotoxin type A (BoNTA) injection for spasmodic dysphonia (SD). BoNTA injection can be performed using (**a**) electromyographic (EMG) guidance or (**b**) direct visualization of the vocal folds using flexible laryngoscopic guidance

between the dose and the response. The typically planned interval between injections is 3–4 months, as the optimal effect of BoNTA injection persists for almost three months. At the visit following an injection, the injection dose and method are adjusted based on the patients' vocal demand, treatment responses, and side effects such as husky voice, aspiration, or dysphagia after the injection. The long-term treatment efficacy of BoNTA injection did not differ between two laterality groups in a previous study, although the treatment interval of alternating unilateral injections was shorter than that of bilateral injections [15, 17]. Patients' age, gender, and VHI scores were correlated with inadequate treatment responses, such as frequent dose changes and shorter intervals between injections [18]. Nevertheless, the mean doses decrease over time, suggesting that bilateral or alternating unilateral BoNTA injections might lead to central nervous system (CNS) network adjustment, enabling a dose reduction over time without the development of tolerance or desensitization [6, 18, 19].

16.1.3 BoNTA Injection Techniques for Adductor SD

BoNTA injections can be administered with EMG guidance or direct visualization of the vocal folds using flexible laryngoscopic guidance. In many cases, EMG localization is considered more straightforward and quicker than laryngoscopic guidance. BoNTA 100 U is reconstituted with 10 mL of 0.9% sodium chloride injection solution, and an appropriate volume is prepared before injection according to the dose. The injection can be administered with the patient sitting or in the supine position. A small amount of xylocaine can be injected into the cricothyroid space. A Teflon-coated 27-gauge EMG needle is percutaneously inserted through the cricothyroid membrane 0.5–1 cm lateral to the midline. The "walking down" technique described in Chap. 6 can be used to quickly identify the inferior border of the thyroid cartilage by palpating the thyroid cartilage while lowering the needle step by step until there is no palpable cartilage. After puncturing the cricothyroid membrane, the needle tip is turned 45–50° laterally and superiorly into the TA muscle. Using flexible laryngoscopic guidance, the level of the cricothyroid membrane and positioning of the needle in the larynx can be determined by observing the mucosal elevation caused by palpating the needle (Fig. 16.2).

For bilateral injection, the needle can be directed superiorly and laterally into the other vocal fold without withdrawing it from the neck. When EMG guidance is used, action potentials indicate placement in the muscle, whereas interference noise indicates that the needle has pene-

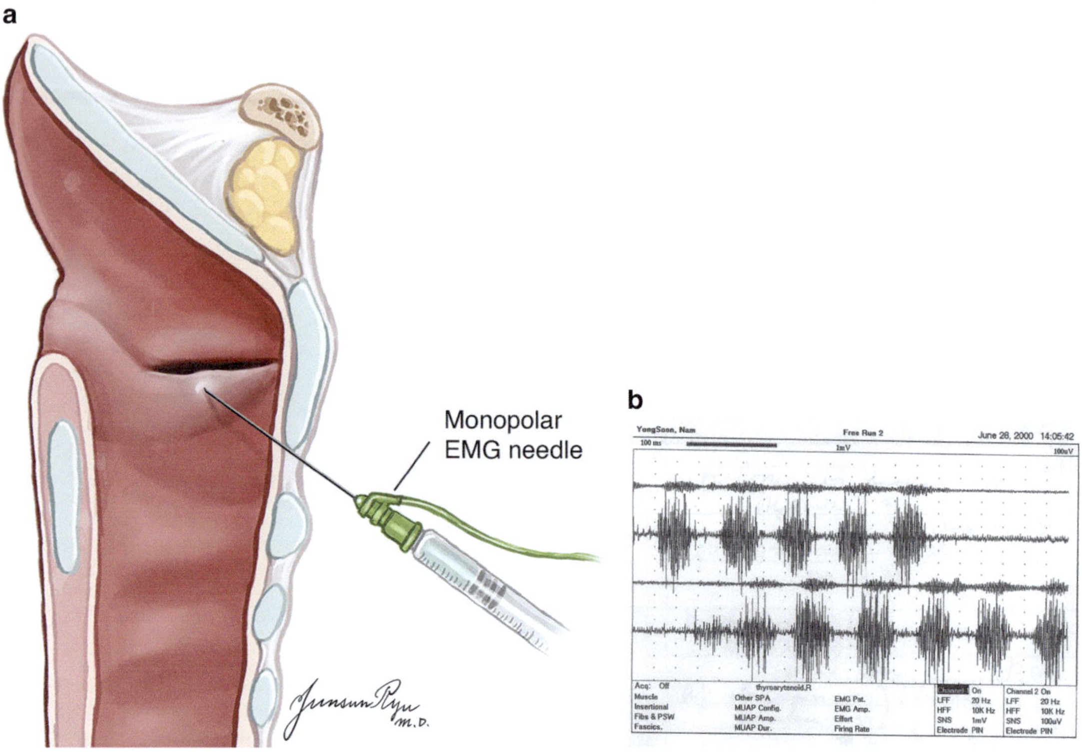

Fig. 16.2 Electromyography (EMG)-guided botulinum neurotoxin type A (BoNTA) injection using the trans-cricothyroid approach. (**a**) Teflon-coated 27-gauge EMG needle was percutaneously inserted through the cricothyroid membrane 0.5–1 cm lateral to the midline. After puncturing the cricothyroid membrane, the needle tip was turned 45–50° laterally and superiorly into the TA muscle. (**b**) BoNTA was then administered after the detection of an EMG signal indicating hyperactivity at the target TA muscle

trated the tracheal lumen [20]. BoNTA is then administered after an EMG signal is detected, indicating hyperactivity at the target TA muscle. Care should be taken to avoid the needle penetrating the airway mucosa because the patients may have the urge to cough and experience dripping of the injected drug if BoNTA is administered with the needle inappropriately placed in the airspace. The patient's next visit is usually determined based on their needs rather than a fixed visit schedule. Patients who are irresponsive to BoNTA injections are treated with a higher dose or subsequent injections at short intervals.

Similar to the technique described above, this procedure can be performed through the thyrohyoid space or mouth. Trans-thyrohyoid and trans-oral approaches are described in Chapters 7 and 5, respectively. Briefly, local anesthesia can be induced by injecting the agent into the skin just above the thyroid notch and deeper into the tissues. The needle is then passed through the midline just above the thyroid notch, directed inferiorly, and visualized as it enters the larynx. It can be directed inferiorly to one side until it can be seen entering the vocal fold where the injection can be administered. The trans-oral approach can be performed by injecting BoNTA through the mouth while directly visualizing the vocal folds using a direct or indirect laryngoscope with a curved needle that can penetrate the vocal folds through the mouth. Similarly, the needle is directed to the vocal folds at the unilateral or bilateral sides, and then the injection can be administered. These two techniques are technically feasible and safe; however, the needle is longer, and the volume withdrawn may not be correctly estimated in these techniques.

16.2 Treatment of Abductor SD

16.2.1 General Principles of BoNTA Injection for Abductor SD

Patients with abductor SD have breathy voice breaks or a continuously breathy voice. Abductor SD can be treated by injecting BoNTA into the posterior cricoarytenoid (PCA) muscle. Unilateral injections do not often adequately mitigate the symptoms of SD, and care should be taken when a bilateral injection is administered because a bilateral injection can also weaken the inspiratory opening by weakening the abduction of the vocal folds or swallowing peristalsis through paralyzing pharyngeal constriction [21]. A dose-escalation protocol with asymmetric bilateral injections has been shown to be effective in treating patients with abductor SD [22]. Flexible laryngoscopy is used to identify the side with dominant abductor activity, which is then injected with 5–10 units, whereas 1.25 units are administered to the other side [1]. Simultaneous, symmetric, bilateral injections of 2.5 units per side have also been reported [21]. If the initial dose is not adequate, the additional toxin can be injected into the dominant PCA muscle until the spams are suppressed. Patients with abductor SD also have decreased adductor muscle activity during phonation, so glottis closure may still be inadequate, although the PCA muscle activity is suppressed.

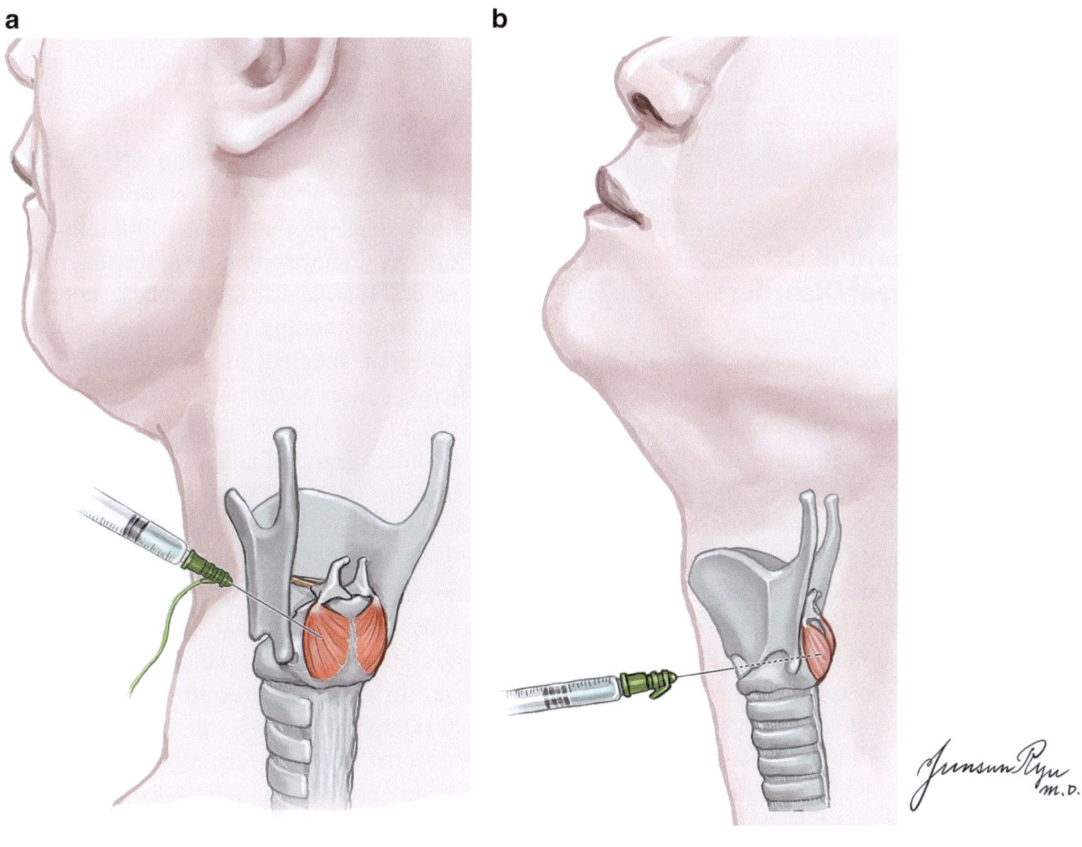

Fig. 16.3 Botulinum neurotoxin type A (BoNTA) injection for abductor spasmodic dysphonia. Lateral (**a**) and (**b**) anterior approaches

16.2.2 BoNTA Injection Techniques for Abductor SD

The PCA muscle is located on the posterior aspect of the larynx, which makes accessing this muscle for an injection technically more complex than treating adductor SD. There are two approaches to injecting BoNTA into the PCA muscle. The first is the "lateral approach" where the larynx is rotated away from the side of injection by depressing the area just medial to the sternocleidomastoid muscle using fingertips and engaging the thyroid ala. The EMG needle is then inserted through the skin 5–10 mm caudal to the cricoid and directed upward and medially to contact the posterior cricoid. The second approach is the "anterior approach" where the needle passes through the cricothyroid membrane, the subglottic airspace, and then the posterior cricoid cartilage until the needle tip is in the PCA muscle. A more lateral approach has also been used, where the needle passes posteriorly along the inner surface of the cricoid without entering the airspace (Fig. 16.3).

16.3 Treatment of Other Laryngeal Disorders

Laryngeal tremor is characterized by rhythmic hyperactivity of the intrinsic or extrinsic laryngeal muscles, resulting in a periodic oscillation of the phonatory apparatus. Tremors of the intrinsic laryngeal musculature occur in 26–53% of patients with SD. BoNTA has been shown to have variable and generally inferior benefits in patients with laryngeal tremors compared with those observed in patients with adductor SD. The most commonly affected muscle complex in laryngeal tremors is the thyroarytenoid/lateral cricoarytenoid (TA/LCA) muscle complex. However, involuntary movement of muscles has been suggested to contribute to the inconsistent efficacy of BoNTA treatment. Patel et al. [23] reported the outcomes of BoNTA treatment for adductor SD, laryngeal tremors, or both [23]. In that study, patients were injected with reconstituted lyophilized BoNTA in the unilateral or bilateral TA/LCA muscle complex using a hollow-bore, 27-gauge Teflon-coated EMG needle with EMG guidance [23]. The injection dose and laterality were adjusted based on patient diary-reported outcomes and preferences with the dual goal of optimizing the time when the patient's voice is normalized and minimizing the breathy period or swallowing adverse effects. Specifically, patients are requested to use a diary to record the grading of the severity of voice breaks (0, no symptoms to 5, voice spasms present 100% of the time) and tremor severity (0, no tremor to 4, can hardly speak). After each BoNTA injection, patients are required to maintain a diary of voice outcomes. BoNTA injections into the TA/LCA complex are an effective treatment for adductor SD, laryngeal tremors, or both; however, the most remarkable effectiveness was observed in patients with tremor-free adductor SD. Defining tremor directionality may facilitate the prognostication of the outcomes of BoNTA injections in patients presenting with tremor components.

Contact granuloma is a relatively rare and benign hypertrophic lesion that occurs posterior to the vocal process due to inflammation that produces granulated tissue at the ulceration sites. Several therapeutic approaches, including voice rest, voice therapy, antibiotics, corticosteroids (injected, inhaled, or parenteral), antireflux therapy, laser treatment, botulinum toxin injection, and surgical removal have been used to treat contact granuloma. However, the condition can recur in 20–90% of patients, irrespective of treatment modalities. Recently, Lee et al. [15] conducted a multicenter study to evaluate the therapeutic efficacy of various modalities and found that botulinum toxin, antireflux treatment, and voice therapy were effective. In contrast, steroid inhalation and surgical removal did not yield significantly different results based on the observations [9]. BoNTA injection was administered to the adductor muscles (2, 3, or 2.5 units into the ipsilateral thyroid arytenoid, lateral cricoarytenoid, or bilateral thyroarytenoid muscles, respectively), and the response rate to the botulinum toxin was 74.2%, whereas the likelihood of a good response to BoNTA was 58.6 times based on simple observation. BoNTA injection is suggested as a second-line treatment for patients for whom the first treatment was not ineffective and could also be used as a first-line treatment depending on the patient's situation and institutional policies.

Key Learning Points:

- Botulinum neurotoxin type A (BoNTA) has been the first-line treatment for patients diagnosed with adductor spasmodic dysphonia (SD).
- Initial administration of low-dose BoNTA injections is effective even in patients with SD.
- Decisions regarding subsequent BoNTA dosing and follow-up should subsequently be made according to the patient's demographics and response to previous injections.
- Although protocols should be individualized for each patient, unilateral injections can be alternated with more long-term efficacy and stability than those with bilateral injections.
- BoNTA doses tend to remain stable over time irrespective of baseline results; however, patient demographics and injection techniques with physicians' experience might affect overall dose stability.
- Injecting BoNTA into the TA/LCA complex is an effective treatment for adductor SD, laryngeal tremors, or both; however, the most significant effect was observed in patients with tremor-free adductor SD.
- BoNTA injection is suggested as a second-line treatment for patients for whom the first treatment was not effective.

References

1. Blitzer A. Spasmodic dysphonia and botulinum toxin: experience from the largest treatment series. Eur J Neurol. 2010;17(Suppl 1):28–30. https://doi.org/10.1111/j.1468-1331.2010.03047.x.
2. Ludlow CL, Adler CH, Berke GS, et al. Research priorities in spasmodic dysphonia. Otolaryngol Head Neck Surg. 2008;139(4):495–505. https://doi.org/10.1016/j.otohns.2008.05.624.
3. Sapienza CM, Walton S, Murry T. Adductor spasmodic dysphonia and muscular tension dysphonia: acoustic analysis of sustained phonation and reading. J Voice. 2000;14(4):502–20. https://doi.org/10.1016/s0892-1997(00)80008-9.
4. Roy N, Mazin A, Awan SN. Automated acoustic analysis of task dependency in adductor spasmodic dysphonia versus muscle tension dysphonia. Laryngoscope. 2014;124(3):718–24. https://doi.org/10.1002/lary.24362.
5. Troung DD, Rontal M, Rolnick M, et al. Double-blind controlled study of botulinum toxin in adductor spasmodic dysphonia. Laryngoscope. 1991;101(6 Pt 1):630–4. https://doi.org/10.1288/00005537-199106000-00010.
6. Blitzer A, Brin MF, Simonyan K, et al. Phenomenology, genetics, and CNS network abnormalities in laryngeal dystonia: a 30-year experience. Laryngoscope 128 Suppl. 2018;1(Suppl 1):S1–s9. https://doi.org/10.1002/lary.27003.
7. Shoffel-Havakuk H, Rosow DE, Lava CX, et al. Common practices in botulinum toxin injection for spasmodic dysphonia treatment: a national survey. Laryngoscope. 2019;129(7):1650–6. https://doi.org/10.1002/lary.27696.
8. Eskander A, Fung K, McBride S, et al. Current practices in the management of adductor spasmodic dysphonia. J Otolaryngol Head Neck Surg. 2010;39(5):622–30.
9. Kim JW, Park JH, Park KN, et al. Treatment efficacy of electromyography versus fiberscopy-guided botulinum toxin injection in adductor spasmodic dysphonia patients: a prospective comparative study. ScientificWorldJournal. 2014;2014:327928. https://doi.org/10.1155/2014/327928.
10. Fulmer SL, Merati AL, Blumin JH. Efficacy of laryngeal botulinum toxin injection: comparison of two techniques. Laryngoscope. 2011;121(9):1924–8. https://doi.org/10.1002/lary.21966.
11. Blitzer A, Brin MF, Stewart CF. Botulinum toxin management of spasmodic dysphonia (laryngeal dystonia): a 12-year experience in more than 900 patients. Laryngoscope. 2015;125(8):1751–7. https://doi.org/10.1002/lary.25273.
12. Rosow DE, Pechman A, Saint-Victor S, et al. Factors influencing botulinum toxin dose instability in spasmodic dysphonia patients. J Voice. 2015;29(3):352–5. https://doi.org/10.1016/j.jvoice.2014.08.011.

13. Dharia I, Bielamowicz S. Unilateral versus bilateral botulinum toxin injections in adductor spasmodic dysphonia in a large cohort. Laryngoscope. 2019; https://doi.org/10.1002/lary.28457.
14. Bielamowicz S, Stager SV, Badillo A, et al. Unilateral versus bilateral injections of botulinum toxin in patients with adductor spasmodic dysphonia. J Voice. 2002;16(1):117–23. https://doi.org/10.1016/s0892-1997(02)00080-2.
15. Lee SJ, Kang MS, Choi HS, et al. Alternating unilateral versus bilateral injections of botulinum toxin for the treatment of adductor spasmodic dysphonia. Otolaryngol Head Neck Surg. 2020;194599820957608 https://doi.org/10.1177/0194599820957608.
16. Bielamowicz S, Ludlow CL. Effects of botulinum toxin on pathophysiology in spasmodic dysphonia. Ann Otol Rhinol Laryngol. 2000;109(2):194–203. https://doi.org/10.1177/000348940010900215.
17. Tang CG, Novakovic D, Mor N, et al. Onabotulinum toxin a dosage trends over time for adductor spasmodic dysphonia: a 15-year experience. Laryngoscope. 2016;126(3):678–81. https://doi.org/10.1002/lary.25551.
18. Kang MS, Lee SJ, Choi HS et al. Factors influencing long-term treatment response to botulinum toxin injection for spasmodic dysphonia. Clin Otolaryngol. 2021;46(2):436–44.
19. Birkent H, Maronian N, Waugh P, et al. Dosage changes in patients with long-term botulinum toxin use for laryngeal dystonia. Otolaryngol Head Neck Surg. 2009;140(1):43–7. https://doi.org/10.1016/j.otohns.2008.10.033.
20. Blitzer A, Crumley RL, Dailey SH, et al. Recommendations of the Neurolaryngology study group on laryngeal electromyography. Otolaryngol Head Neck Surg. 2009;140(6):782–93. https://doi.org/10.1016/j.otohns.2009.01.026.
21. Klein AM, Stong BC, Wise J, et al. Vocal outcome measures after bilateral posterior cricoarytenoid muscle botulinum toxin injections for abductor spasmodic dysphonia. Otolaryngol Head Neck Surg. 2008;139(3):421–3. https://doi.org/10.1016/j.otohns.2008.06.013.
22. Woodson G, Hochstetler H, Murry T. Botulinum toxin therapy for abductor spasmodic dysphonia. J Voice. 2006;20(1):137–43. https://doi.org/10.1016/j.jvoice.2005.03.008.
23. Patel PN, Kabagambe EK, Starkweather JC, et al. Outcomes of Onabotulinum toxin a treatment for adductor spasmodic dysphonia and laryngeal tremor. JAMA Otolaryngol Head Neck Surg. 2018;144(4):293–9. https://doi.org/10.1001/jamaoto.2017.3088.

17 Vocal Fold Steroid Injection

Chi-Te Wang

Abstract

In the modern era of minimally invasive surgery and in-office procedures, vocal fold steroid injection (VFSI) is a valuable and indispensable tool for phonosurgeons in their gearbox. Clinical indications include vocal nodules, polyps, mucus retention cysts, Reinke's edema, scar, and postoperative fibrosis. With the advancement of endoscopic technology, VFSI can be easily performed via trans-oral, trans-nasal, and percutaneous approaches. Adequate laryngeal anesthesia is the key to a smooth procedure, which also requires continual practice and great patience. Most adverse events after VFSI, including hematoma, deposition of triamcinolone, and vocal atrophy, are self-limited without irreversible sequel. Careful and precise placement of needle superficial to vocal ligament, and injecting minimal amount of steroid helps to avoid these adverse events. Adjuvant voice therapy is encouraged to lower the recurrence rate after VFSI.

C.-T. Wang (✉)
Department of Otolaryngology Head and Neck Surgery, Far Eastern Memorial Hospital, Taipei, Taiwan

Keywords

Office procedures · Nodules · Polyp · Cyst · Reinke's edema · Scar · Fibrosis

17.1 Evolving History of Vocal Fold Steroid Injection (VFSI)

The first recognized literature regarding vocal fold steroid injection (VFSI) was published by Yanagihara et al. in 1964 [1]. The authors described trans-oral injection of prednisolone or dexamethasone for benign vocal fold disorders, which was performed in the office using indirect mirror for visual guidance. Their protocol consisted of 2–3 injections at an interval of 3 days, with 62.5 ~ 79.6% effective rates. Unfortunately, this article did not receive proper attention because of the growing popularity of microsurgery under general anesthesia. Nevertheless, a few studies applied percutaneous intralesional steroid injection for laryngeal stenosis [2, 3], sarcoidosis, systemic lupus erythematosus, and Wegener's granulomatosis [4–6]. Other related studies suggested steroid injection after microsurgical removal of benign vocal fold structural lesions to reduce scar formation during the healing process [7, 8].

VFSI as the primary treatment modality for benign vocal fold lesions was not widely accepted until the 2000s. Tateya et al. applied flexible fiberscope to ensure precise injection of triam-

© Springer Nature Singapore Pte Ltd. 2021
B.-J. Lee et al. (eds.), *Vocal Fold Injection*, https://doi.org/10.1007/978-981-16-3303-4_17

cinolone for patients of vocal nodules and Reinke's edema [9, 10]. Since then, a surge of studies demonstrated that VFSI can be effective to treat other benign vocal fold lesions, such as polyp, cyst, scar, and granuloma [11–13]. With technical advancement of a distal-chip flexible endoscope and fiber-based laser (e.g., KTP laser), another paradigm shift toward office-based laryngeal procedures under local anesthesia has gradually taken place in the past decades [14, 15].

17.2 Mechanisms of Steroid Injection for Benign Vocal Lesions

It is well known that pharmacological effects of corticosteroids are quite complex (e.g., carbohydrate, protein, and lipid metabolism; increased hepatic capacity for gluconeogenesis; enhanced catabolic actions upon muscle, skin, lymphoid, adipose and connective tissues; immunomodulation via various cytokines on lymphocytes and macrophages.) [16]; herein, the mechanism of corticosteroid on benign vocal lesions are commonly attributed to its "anti-inflammatory effects" without detailed investigation. Tracing back the history, Coleman, et al. noted a delay in the inflammatory and neovascular responses following treatment of triamcinolone on the microflap wounds of 15 dogs [17]. A subsequent study demonstrated a trend of decreased COX-2 gene expression by prophylactic intralaryngeal triamcinolone acetonide injection after acute phonotrauma [18], despite the result did not reach statistical significance.

According to the studies from keloid and granulation tissue [19, 20], the profound inhibitory effects of corticosteroid on fibroblast and collagen synthesis contribute part of the mechanism of vocal fold steroid injection. In the histological study conducted by Campagnolo, et al., rabbits treated by dexamethasone revealed significantly decreased rates and amount of collagen deposition during the acute healing process (within 7 days) of surgically injured vocal folds [21]. A later study also demonstrated that exogenous dexamethasone can significantly reduce fibroblast proliferation and TGF-ß-induced collagen synthesis, in a dose-dependent fashion [22]. Considering that repeated vibration of vocal folds could result in epithelial barrier dysfunction [23], another possible mechanism of VFSI might be related to the effects of steroid on epithelial cell tight junction formation [24] or the regulation of proinflammatory cytokines [25].

Although the actual mechanism of VFSI is not fully understood, intralesional corticosteroid might take effect across the whole inflammatory stages, i.e., reduces capillary permeability immediately after acute phonotrauma; downregulates the cytokines during the recruitment of inflammatory cells; and reduces collagen synthesis fibroblast activity to prevent scar/fibrosis formation. Following diagram summarized the current understanding of the mechanism of intralesional corticosteroid injection on benign vocal fold lesions (Fig. 17.1).

17.3 Techniques and Injection Routes of VFSI

Several different approaches for performing VFSI have been proposed in the published literature, including: (1) trans-oral approach guided by flexible fiberscope [1, 9, 10]; (2) trans-oral injection guided by rigid 70-degree telescope [11]; (3) trans-cutaneous via cricothyroid membrane guided by flexible endoscope [12, 26, 27], and (4) trans-nasal approach via the working channel of distal-chip flexible endoscope [28]. We will illustrate our preferred two approaches (i.e., trans-oral with rigid telescope and trans-nasal approach via the working channel) in this section.

Trans-oral approach is the most natural route to access the larynx and vocal folds; nevertheless, it requires a long-learning curve to be familiar with the long and curved injection needle. Moreover, adequate anesthesia of oropharynx and larynx is a prerequisite of smooth and successful injection procedure, which also requires tremendous patience and experience to be mastered. Following years of practice, our protocol of laryngeal anesthesia for trans-oral injection includes the following steps:

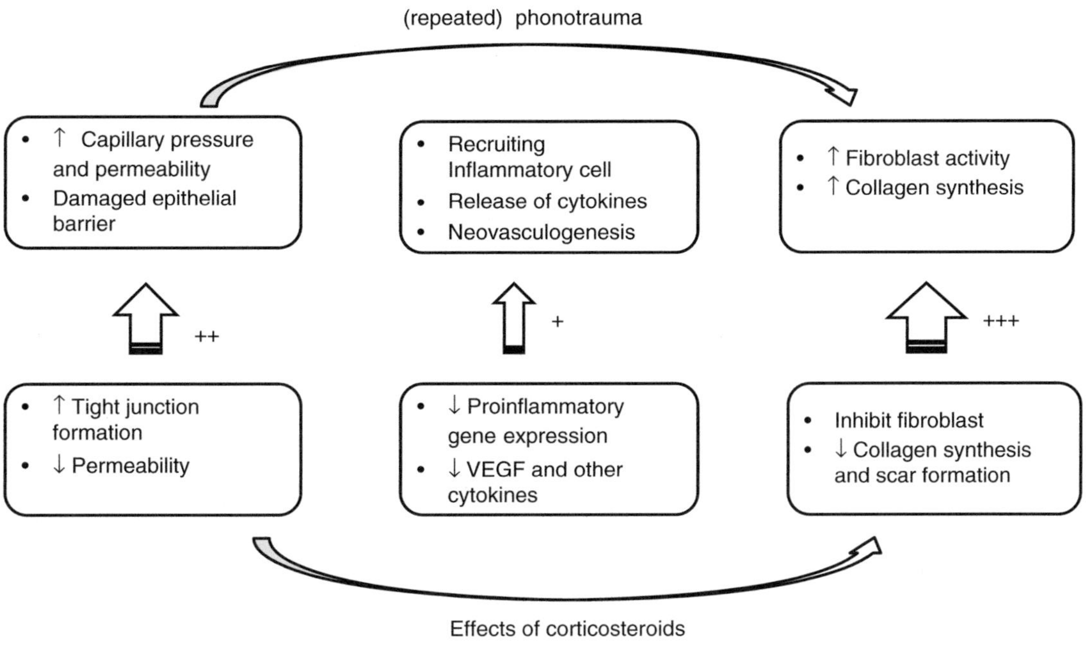

Note: "+, ++, +++" represent strength of evidences

Fig. 17.1 Proposed mechanism of corticosteroids across different stages of phonotrauma

1. Topical spray 2% lidocaine over soft palate, uvula, tonsillar fossa, and posterior pharyngeal wall.
2. Topical spray 10% lidocaine over the base of tongue and gradually proceeds deeper toward vallecula.
3. Laryngeal gargle of 2% lidocaine (4~5 ml). We usually ask the patient to phonate "ee" sound and drip 0.5–1.0 ml lidocaine at a time, followed by a short cough to prevent aspiration.

Adequate laryngeal anesthesia can be confirmed by the absence of laryngeal adductor reflex. Usually, operators can have a 5–10 minutes "window" to perform the injection procedures. Surgeons should always keep in mind the maximum dose of lidocaine (i.e., 4.5 mg/kg) and pay attention to early sign of lidocaine overdose/intoxication [29].

We usually use the nondominant hand to hold a rigid 70-degree telescope and ask the patient to pull his/her own tongue out (Fig. 17.2). Alternatively, the surgeon can ask an assistant (e.g., resident doctor) to hold a trans-nasal flexible fiberscope for visualization, and pull out the patient's tongue by the surgeon himself while inject steroid trans-orally [9]. In such way, the procedure may require additional anesthesia to the nasal cavity and may cause irritation/discomfort when inserting and manipulating trans-nasal endoscope. We preferred a curved injection apparatus with a disposable needle (Model 16–50050, Medtronic Xomed Jacksonville, Florida, USA). In cases when the prefixed angle of this device is not suitable, e.g., higher larynx or shorter neck, a malleable injection needle can be applied alternatively (Fig. 17.3).

For patients who cannot tolerate the above trans-oral approach, our second choice would be trans-nasal approach using the operating channel of a flexible endoscope (Fig. 17.4) [28]. Compared with percutaneous or trans-oral approaches guided by trans-nasal endoscope, the most clear advantage of this approach is that it does not require additional puncture of anterior neck skin, neither does it need to pull the patients tongue out. Anesthesia procedure

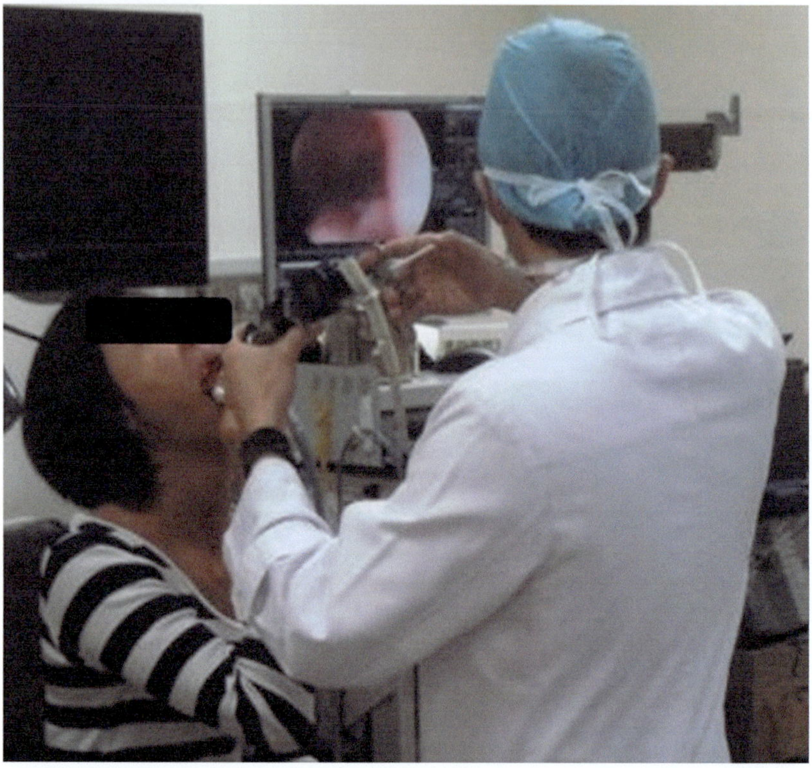

Fig. 17.2 Trans-oral VFSI performed as a single surgeon procedure

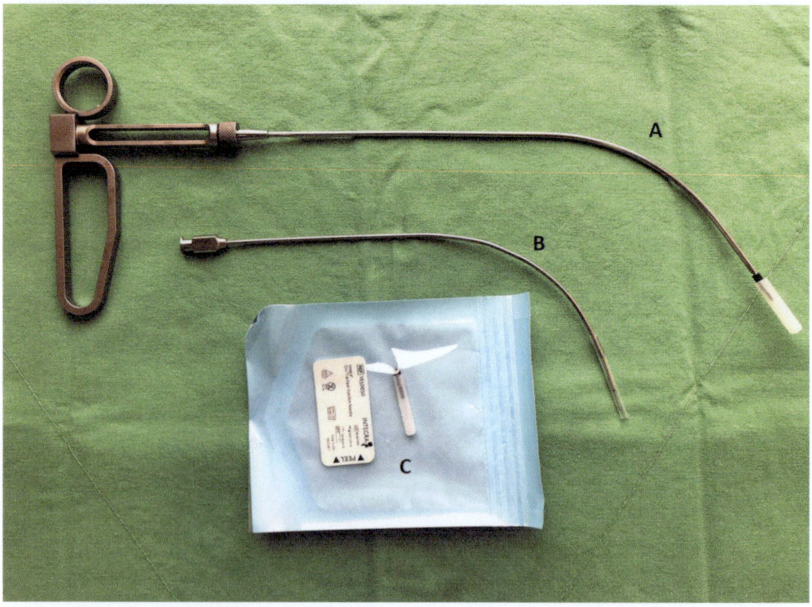

Fig. 17.3 Equipment for trans-oral VFSI. Injection apparatus (**A**) with disposable needle tip (**C**). Malleable injection needle (**B**)

start from nasal packing with cotton pledget soaked with epinephrine and xylocaine. Laryngeal gargle can be performed in similar ways by inserting a spraying tube (Olympus PW-6P-1) via the working channel. We used a flexible endoscopic injection apparatus (Olympus NM-101C-0427), which includes a reusable metallic external sheath (MAJ-655)

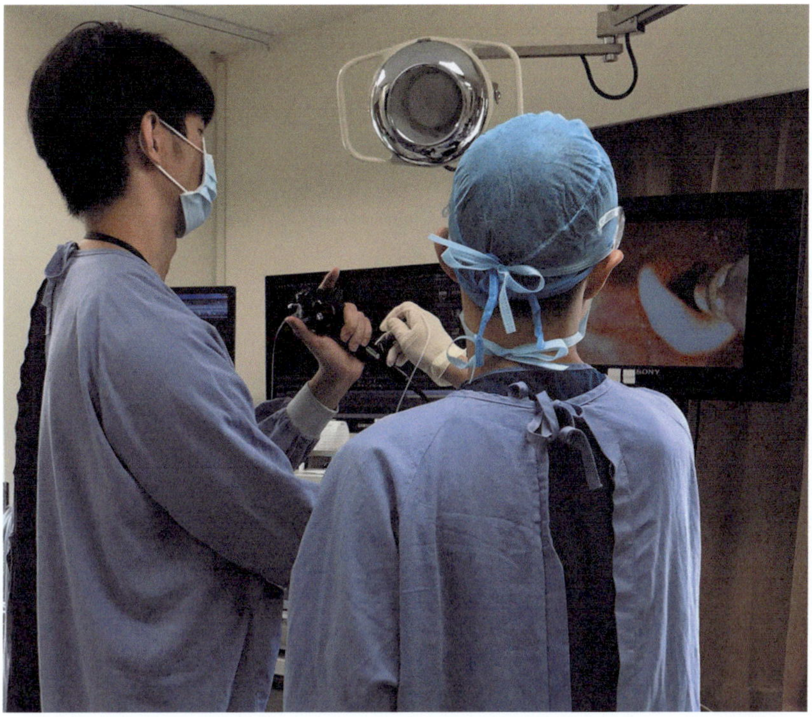

Fig. 17.4 Trans-nasal approach of VFSI. The assistant handle the flexible fiberscope while the surgeon insert and operate instruments via the working channel

and a disposable flexible needle with a 27G tip (MAJ-656) (Fig. 17.5).

No matter what approaches, surgeons should inject steroid into the superficial lamina propria immediately adjacent to the lesion (e.g., nodules or polyp), and the needle tip should stay as superficial as possible, away from vocal ligament and vocalis muscle. We usually inject 0.1–0.2 ml of steroid in each lesion. Care should be taken not to penetrate through the upper and lower lip of vocal folds to avoid leakage of injected steroids. Diffuse infiltration of steroid over the superficial lamina propria is not recommended, with the only exception in cases of Reinke's edema.

17.4 Indications for VFSI

A previous systematic review and meta-analysis identified several voice disorders suitable for VFSI, including Reinke's edema, vocal nodules, polyp, cyst, granuloma, and vocal scar [13]. Because all the earlier studies were based on pre-post study design without a comparison/control group, we conducted the first comparative study of VFSI to further validate its effectiveness [30]. Lesion size reduced for 39% and 46%, 1 and 2 month after VFSI, respectively. In comparison, lesion size reduced for 6% and 24%, 1 and 2 months following vocal hygiene education, which showed significant statistical differences ($p < 0.05$, t tests).

In our hands, the most frequent indications for VFSI were vocal nodules, polyps, and cysts. Details of outcome improvements can be found in our previous publication [31]. Clinical experience showed that VFSI works well in soft/early vocal nodules with 70–80% response rate (improved voice quality and decreased lesion size) (Fig. 17.6). Thick, fibrotic nodules may also benefit from VFSI, though less likely to resolve completely.

Compared with nodules, the clinical application of VFSI in vocal polyps shall be more selective based on its various presentation. From our experience, favorable cases are translucent, wide-based, and recently onset polyps (Fig. 17.7). In contrast, we prefer KTP laser procedures (with or without polypectomy) for pedunculated and hemorrhagic polyps [32–34]. For long-standing,

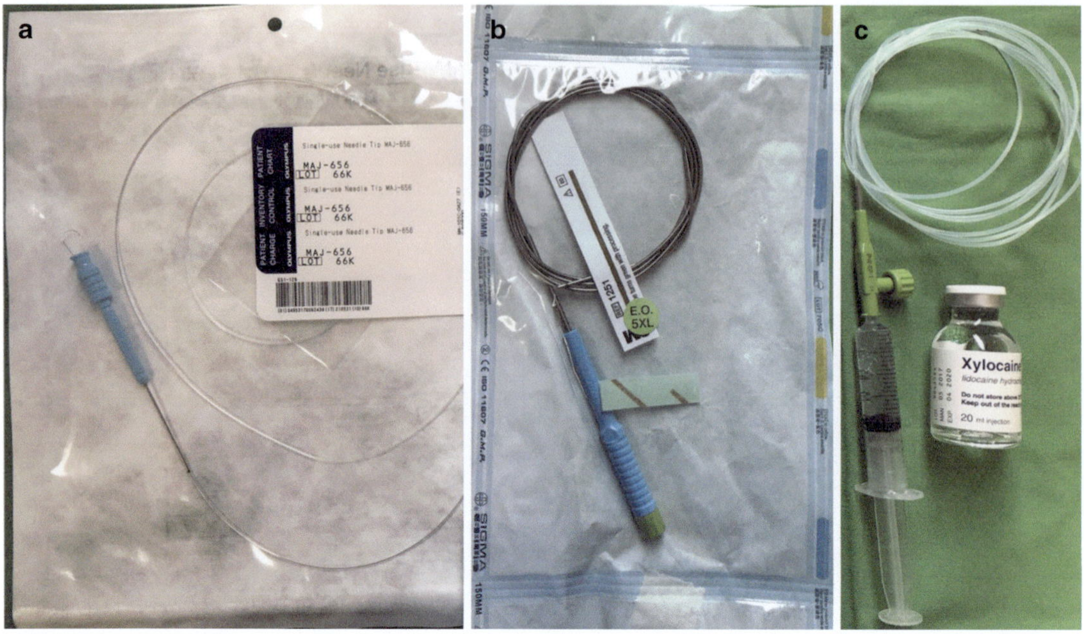

Fig. 17.5 Equipment for trans-nasal VFSI. (**a**) 27G Flexible injection needle, (**b**) metallic sheath, (**c**) flexible tube for spraying local anesthetics

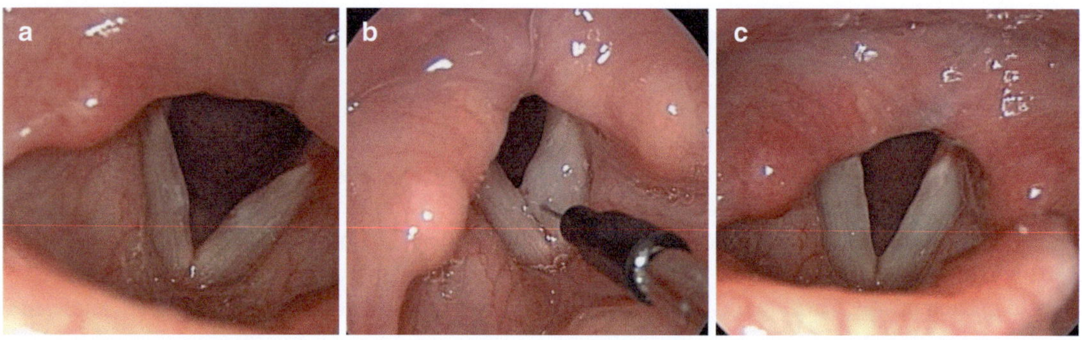

Fig. 17.6 (**a**) Vocal nodules in a 42-year-old female patient; (**b**) trans-oral VFSI; (**c**) lesion resolved after VFSI

fibrotic, and huge polyps, VFSI has minimal effects and phonomicrosurgery remains the gold standard of treatment.

VFSI can be an alternative treatment for mucus retention cyst, especially for patients not suitable for microsurgery because of personal consideration (e.g., afraid of general anesthesia) or difficult anatomy for direct suspension laryngoscope. In a recent study, 48 out of 57 (84%) cases of mucus retention cyst exhibited substantial lesion resolution after VFSI (Fig. 17.8), and the voice outcome was significantly better than age- and sex- matched patients receiving only conservative managements [35]. Possible explanations of the observed effectiveness of VFSI for vocal cysts include: (1) direct puncture of cyst wall and drainage of cystic content; (2) anti-inflammatory effect of steroid re-opens the mucus excretory route; and (3) steroid might cause synechia/adhesion of cyst wall and prevent re-accumulation of mucus, similar to sclerosing therapy of neck cysts [36].

Previous studies had reported the application of VFSI in cases of Reinke's edema [9, 27]. Nevertheless, Reinke's edema comprised a wide range of clinical presentation from minimal

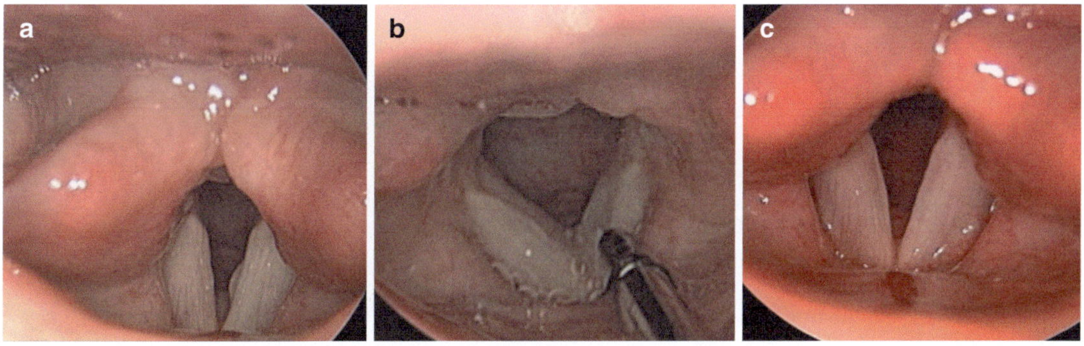

Fig. 17.7 (**a**) vocal polyp in a 31-year-old female patient; (**b**) trans-oral VFSI; (**c**) lesion resolved after VFSI

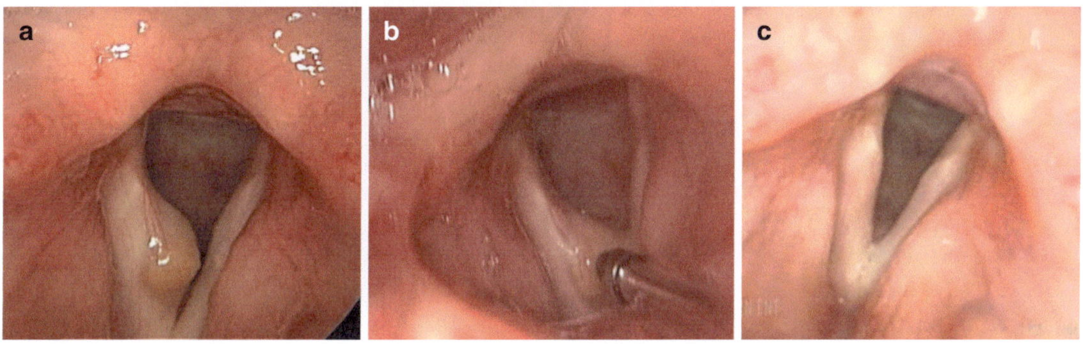

Fig. 17.8 (**a**) Mucus retention cyst of right vocal fold in 53-year-old male patient; (**b**) trans-oral VFSI; (**c**) lesion resolved

edema to profound deformity of vocal fold due to the accumulation of polypoid content (i.e., polypoid corditis). The application of VFSI might be beneficial for mild disease/early stage of Reinke's edema (Yonekawa type I) [37], whereas microsurgery should be the treatment of choice for later stages of polypoid corditis (type II or III).

Another potential application of VFSI is vocal fold fibrosis and scar. Because there is no standard treatment so far, VFSI represent a reasonable trial option owing to its antifibrotic effects [21, 38]. A small case series [39] reported improvement of voice outcomes following a single in-office VFSI for mild to moderate scar, which were not resulted from prior microsurgery [39]. A recent study further documented that VFSI can be an adjuvant treatment for fibrotic change following phonomicrosurgery. The results showed that 76% of postoperative vocal fold fibrosis presented with better mucosal wave, improved voice quality, and less dysphonic symptoms after 1–2 courses of VFSI [40]. Other potential indications of VFSI include subglottic stenosis [41, 42], and vocal process granuloma [11, 43].

17.5 Adverse Events after VFSI

The most commonly encountered adverse events after VFSI are hematoma, deposition of injected material, and atrophic change of vocal folds [13, 31]. The reported incidence rates of vocal hematoma after VFSI ranged from 1 to 20% [12, 27, 31]. Rates of whitish plaque deposition of the injected triamcinolone varied from 2.5% to nearly 100% [26, 27, 44] (Fig. 17.9). Atrophic change of vocal folds ranged from 1 to 5% in various published series [26, 31]. Such a discrepancy of reported incidence rates of adverse events following VFSI can be related to the timing of

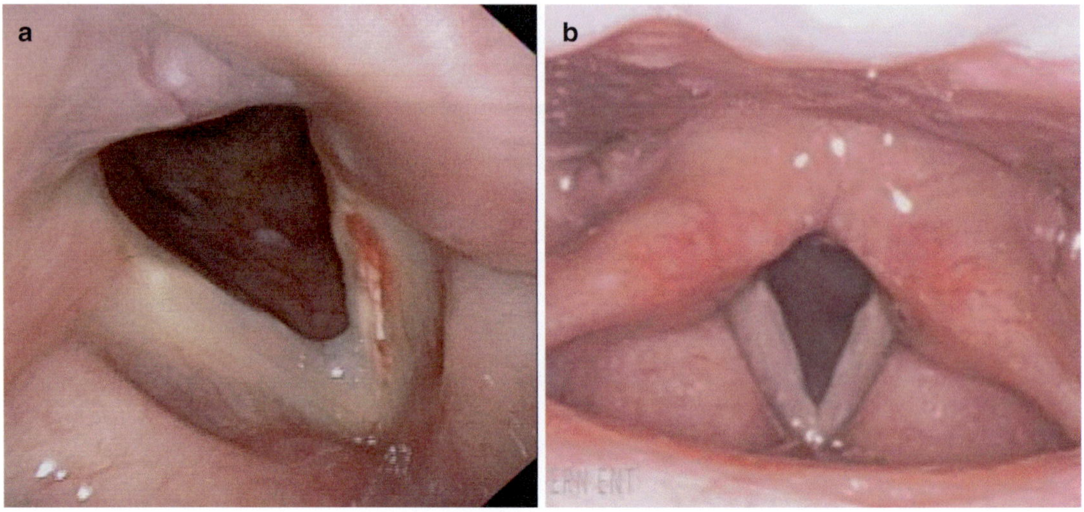

Fig. 17.9 (**a**) Whitish plaque deposition of triamcinolone acetonide, which gradually absorbed after 6 weeks (**b**)

follow-up visits. The chance to observe hematoma and deposition after VFSI would be higher if the patients return to the clinics shortly after VFSI (e.g. 1–2 weeks).

Vocal atrophy is probably the most worried adverse events after VFSI. A previous study proposed that most cases resulted from mucus gland atrophy [11]; however, we do occasionally observe bowing of vocal folds with sunken ventricle, indicating atrophy of lamina propria and musculature (Fig. 17.10). Nevertheless, our practice in the past decade confirmed that nearly all adverse events, including atrophic change of vocal folds, gradually recovered within 4–6 weeks. We have not encountered long-standing, nonreversible sequel so far.

In order to balance between the pros (longer duration) and cons (higher chance of deposition and plaque formation) of triamcinolone acetonide, we prefer to inject 1:1 mixture of triamcinolone and dexamethasone as our routine protocol [28, 45]. Meanwhile, care should be taken to stay away from vocal ligament during injection to avoid atrophic change, especially in bottom-up percutaneous injection routes (e.g. injection via cricothyroid membrane). In addition, surgeon should inject a minimal amount of steroid (0.1~0.2 ml) and avoid diffuse infiltration of steroid within the lamina propria. Finally, 2–3 days of voice rest after VFSI is enough for most cases. A longer period of voice rest, e.g., 1–2 weeks, might result in delayed recovery owing to disuse atrophy.

17.6 Recurrence of Vocal Lesions after VFSI

It is well understood that most benign vocal lesions are resulted from chronic overuse or misuse of voice. Not surprisingly, lesion recurrence after VFSI is frequently encountered. Lee et al. reported 20 out of 84 patients (23.8%) with lesion recurrence, 12 months after VFSI [45]. The average interval to recurrence was 8.5 months and was associated with voice abuse and higher vocal demand. Another study followed 139 patients receiving VFSI via telephone interview for 2 years [46]. Treatment failure was defined by (1) recurring symptoms with VHI-10 > 10 points; or (2) receiving secondary interventions (i.e., repeated VFSI or microsurgery). The cumulative failure rates following VFSI were 12%, 17%, 24%, and 32%, at 6, 12, 18, and 24 months, respectively. Accordingly, patient should be informed about the high recurrence rates prior to VFSI and should receive postoperative voice therapy.

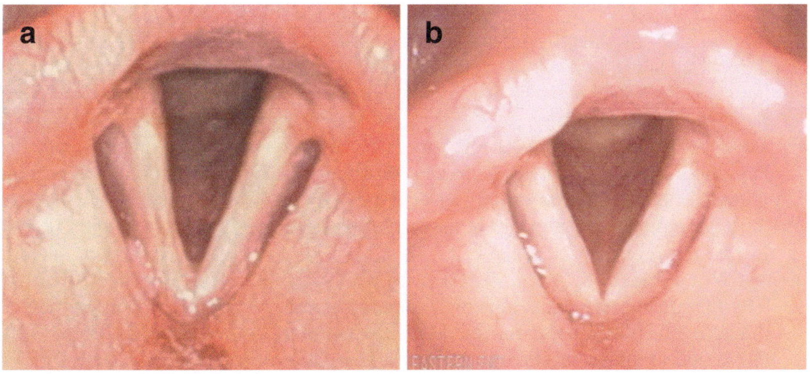

Fig. 17.10 (**a**) Atrophic change of lamina propria and vocalis muscles after VFSI in a 40-year-old female patient, which recovered spontaneously after 1 month (**b**)

Key Learning Points:

- Vocal fold steroid injection (VFSI) is an effective treatment option for vocal nodules, polyps, mucus retention cysts, Reinke's edema, scar, and fibrosis.
- VFSI can be performed via trans-oral, trans-nasal, and percutaneous approaches.
- Adverse events of VFSI include vocal hematoma, deposition of triamcinolone, and vocal atrophy. Most adverse events resolve spontaneously without long-term sequel.
- Recurrence following VFSI is not uncommon, and voice therapy should be encouraged after VFSI.

References

1. Yanagihara N, Azuma F, Koike Y, Honjo I, Imanishi Y. Intracordal injection of dexamethasone. Pract Otorhinolaryngol. 1964;57:496–500.
2. Rosen G, Vered IY. Triamcinolone acetonide injection for laryngeal stenosis. J Laryngol Otol. 1975;89:1043–6.
3. Gnanapragasam A. Intralesional steroids in conservative management of subglottic stenosis of the larynx. Int Surg. 1979;64:63–7.
4. Krespi YP, Mitrani M, Husain S, Meltzer CJ. Treatment of laryngeal sarcoidosis with intralesional steroid injection. Ann Otol Rhinol Laryngol. 1987;96:713–5.
5. Teitel AD, MacKenzie CR, Stern R, Paget SA. Laryngeal involvement in systemic lupus erythematosus. Semin Arthritis Rheum. 1992;22:203–14.
6. Gulati SP, Sachdeva OP, Sachdeva A, Singh U. Wegener's granulomatosis: a case with laryngeal involvement. Indian J Chest Dis Allied Sci. 1997;39:125–8.
7. Bouchayer M, Cornut G. Microsurgery for benign lesions of the vocal folds. Ear Nose Throat J. 1988;67:446–9.
8. Courey MS, Gardner GM, Stone RE, Ossoff RH. Endoscopic vocal fold microflap: a three-year experience. Ann Otol Rhinol Laryngol. 1995;104:267–73.
9. Tateya I, Omori K, Kojima H, Hirano S, Kaneko K, Ito J. Steroid injection for Reinke's edema using fiberoptic laryngeal surgery. Acta Otolaryngol. 2003;123:417–20.
10. Tateya I, Omori K, Kojima H, Hirano S, Kaneko K, Ito J. Steroid injection to vocal nodules using fiberoptic laryngeal surgery under topical anesthesia. Eur Arch Otorhinolaryngol. 2004;261:489–92.
11. Mortensen M, Woo P. Office steroid injections of the larynx. Laryngoscope. 2006;116:1735–9.
12. Hsu YB, Lan MC, Chang SY. Percutaneous corticosteroid injection for vocal fold polyp. Arch Otolaryngol Head Neck Surg. 2009;135:776–80.
13. Wang CT, Liao LJ, Cheng PW, Lo WC, Lai MS. Intralesional steroid injection for benign vocal fold disorders: a systematic review and meta-analysis. Laryngoscope. 2013;123:197–203.
14. Shah MD, Johns MM. Office-based procedures in laryngology. In: Johnson JT, Rosen CA, eds. Bailey's head & neck surgery - otolaryngology. Lippincott William & Wilkins; 2013. pp. 1078–1090.
15. Shoffel-Havakuk H, Sadoughi B, Sulica L, Johns MM, 3rd. In-office procedures for the treatment of benign vocal fold lesions in the awake patient: A contemporary review. Laryngoscope 2018.
16. Campagnolo AM, Tsuji DH, Sennes LU, Imamura R. Steroid injection in chronic inflammatory vocal fold disorders, literature review. Braz J Otorhinolaryngol. 2008;74:926–32.
17. Coleman JR Jr, Smith S, Reinisch L, et al. Histomorphometric and laryngeal videostroboscopic analysis of the effects of corticosteroids on microflap healing in the dog larynx. Ann Otol Rhinol Laryngol. 1999;108:119–27.

18. Hall JE, Suehiro A, Branski RC, Garrett CG, Rousseau B. Modulation of inflammatory and profibrotic signaling in a rabbit model of acute phonotrauma using triamcinolone. Otolaryngol Head Neck Surg. 2012;147:302–7.
19. Meisler N, Keefer KA, Ehrlich HP, Yager DR, Myers-Parrelli J, Cutroneo KR. Dexamethasone abrogates the fibrogenic effect of transforming growth factor-beta in rat granuloma and granulation tissue fibroblasts. J Invest Dermatol. 1997;108:285–9.
20. Wu WS, Wang FS, Yang KD, Huang CC, Kuo YR. Dexamethasone induction of keloid regression through effective suppression of VEGF expression and keloid fibroblast proliferation. J Invest Dermatol. 2006;126:1264–71.
21. Campagnolo AM, Tsuji DH, Sennes LU, Imamura R, Saldiva PH. Histologic study of acute vocal fold wound healing after corticosteroid injection in a rabbit model. Ann Otol Rhinol Laryngol. 2010;119:133–9.
22. Zhou H, Sivasankar M, Kraus DH, Sandulache VC, Amin M, Branski RC. Glucocorticoids regulate extracellular matrix metabolism in human vocal fold fibroblasts. Laryngoscope. 2011;121:1915–9.
23. Rousseau B, Suehiro A, Echemendia N, Sivasankar M. Raised intensity phonation compromises vocal fold epithelial barrier integrity. Laryngoscope. 2011;121:346–51.
24. Zettl KS, Sjaastad MD, Riskin PM, Parry G, Machen TE, Firestone GL. Glucocorticoid-induced formation of tight junctions in mouse mammary epithelial cells in vitro. Proc Natl Acad Sci U S A. 1992;89:9069–73.
25. Aveleira CA, Lin CM, Abcouwer SF, Ambrosio AF, Antonetti DA. TNF-alpha signals through PKCzeta/NF-kappaB to alter the tight junction complex and increase retinal endothelial cell permeability. Diabetes. 2010;59:2872–82.
26. Lee SH, Yeo JO, Choi JIet al. Local steroid injection via the cricothyroid membrane in patients with a vocal nodule. Arch Otolaryngol Head Neck Surg 2011; 137:1011–1016.
27. Woo JH, Kim DY, Kim JW, Oh EA, Lee SW. Efficacy of percutaneous vocal fold injections for benign laryngeal lesions: prospective multicenter study. Acta Otolaryngol. 2011;131:1326–32.
28. Wang CT, Lai MS, Liao LJ, Lo WC, Cheng PW. Transnasal endoscopic steroid injection: a practical and effective alternative treatment for benign vocal fold disorders. Laryngoscope. 2013;123:1464–8.
29. Rosen CA, Simpson CB. Operative techniques in laryngology. New York: Springer; 2008.
30. Wang CT, Liao LJ, Lai MS, Cheng PW. Comparison of benign lesion regression following vocal fold steroid injection and vocal hygiene education. Laryngoscope. 2014;124:510–5.
31. Wang CT, Lai MS, Hsiao TY. Comprehensive outcome researches of Intralesional steroid injection on benign vocal fold lesions. J Voice. 2015;29:578–87.
32. Wang CT, Huang TW, Liao LJ, Lo WC, Lai MS, Cheng PW. Office-based potassium titanyl phosphate laser-assisted endoscopic vocal polypectomy. JAMA Otolaryngol Head Neck Surg. 2013;139:610–6.
33. Wang CT, Liao LJ, Huang TW, Lo WC, Cheng PW. Comparison of treatment outcomes of transnasal vocal fold polypectomy versus microlaryngoscopic surgery. Laryngoscope. 2015;125:1155–60.
34. Lin YH, Wang CT, Lin FC, Liao LJ, Lo WC, Cheng PW. Treatment outcomes and adverse events following in-office Angiolytic laser with or without concurrent polypectomy for vocal fold polyps. JAMA Otolaryngol Head Neck Surg. 2018;144:222–30.
35. Wu PH, Cheng PW, Lin FC, Wang CT. Intralesional steroid injection as an alternative treatment for 57 patients of vocal fold mucus retention cysts. Clin Otolaryngol. 2018;43:1375–8.
36. Kim MG, Kim SG, Lee JH, Eun YG, Yeo SG. The therapeutic effect of OK-432 (picibanil) sclerotherapy for benign neck cysts. Laryngoscope. 2008;118:2177–81.
37. Yonekawa H. A clinical study of Reinke's edema. Auris Nasus Larynx. 1988;15:57–78.
38. Mortensen M. Laryngeal steroid injection for vocal fold scar. Curr Opin Otolaryngol Head Neck Surg. 2010;18:487–91.
39. Young WG, Hoffman MR, Koszewski IJ, Whited CW, Ruel BN, Dailey SH. Voice outcomes following a single office-based steroid injection for vocal fold scar. Otolaryngol Head Neck Surg. 2016;155:820–8.
40. Hsu YC, Liao LJ, Huang TW, Wang CT. Assessment of patient outcomes after adjuvant vocal fold steroid injection for fibrosis after microlaryngeal surgery. JAMA Otolaryngol Head Neck Surg. 2019;145:811–6.
41. Hoffman MR, Coughlin AR, Dailey SH. Serial office-based steroid injections for treatment of idiopathic subglottic stenosis. Laryngoscope. 2017;127:2475–81.
42. Bertelsen C, Shoffel-Havakuk H, O'Dell K, Johns MM, 3rd, Reder LS. Serial in-office intralesional steroid injections in airway stenosis. JAMA Otolaryngol Head Neck Surg; 2018.
43. Wang CT, Lai MS, Lo WC, Liao LJ, Cheng PW. Intralesional steroid injection: an alternative treatment option for vocal process granuloma in ten patients. Clin Otolaryngol. 2013;38:77–81.
44. Andrade Filho PA, Rosen CA. Vocal fold plaque following triamcinolone injection. Ear Nose Throat J. 2003;82:908–11.
45. Wang CT, Lai MS, Cheng PW. Long-term surveillance following Intralesional steroid injection for benign vocal fold lesions. JAMA Otolaryngol Head Neck Surg. 2017;143:589–94.
46. Lee SW, Park KN. Long-term efficacy of percutaneous steroid injection for treating benign vocal fold lesions: a prospective study. Laryngoscope. 2016;126:2315–9.

18 Vocal Fold Growth Factor Injection

Shigeru Hirano

Abstract

Growth factors are used for regeneration of several organs targeting various refractory diseases. Basic fibroblast growth factor (bFGF) and hepatocyte growth factor (HGF) have been proven to have regenerative effects on the vocal fold mucosa, and to be useful for the treatment of vocal fold scar, sulcus, and atrophy. The vocal fold becomes thin and/or stiff in these pathologies due to excessive collagen deposition and decrease of hyaluronic acid (HA) in the lamina propria of the vocal fold. The growth factors have strong effects of increasing production of HA and decreasing collagen production from vocal fold fibroblasts, which in turn leads to better vibratory properties. Repeated intracordal injection of the growth factors has proved regenerative effects for the vocal fold scar and aged atrophy in animal models. Clinical trials have also indicated positive effects on the vocal fold function in terms of improvement of vibratory amplitude, glottal competence, aerodynamic, and acoustic measures for the patients with vocal fold scar, sulcus, and atrophy.

S. Hirano (✉)
Department of Otolaryngology Head and Neck Surgery, Kyoto Prefectural University of Medicine, Kyoto, Japan
e-mail: hirano@koto.kpu-m.ac.jp

Keywords

Fibroblast growth factor · hepatocyte growth factor · vocal fold atrophy · vocal fold scar sulcus vocalis · intracordal injection regeneration

18.1 Basic Fibroblast Growth Factor

18.1.1 Biological Activity on Wound Healing

Basic fibroblast growth factor was first found as a naturally occurring protein with strong potency of angiogenesis, and then has proved to contribute in organogenesis, wound healing, and regeneration. The bFGF is a stimulant of fibroblast for migration, proliferation, and mitogenesis. It also affects cell function of fibroblast. For example, it was revealed that bFGF increases production of hyaluronic acid (HA) from skin fibroblasts, and it was also demonstrated that bFGF downregulates gene expression of type I collagen in gingival fibroblasts [1, 2]. Collagen matrix gel study showed less contraction of the gel by addition of bFGF [3]. An animal study indicated decrease of granulation during early wound healing of rat skin incisional wounds by intradermal injection

© Springer Nature Singapore Pte Ltd. 2021
B.-J. Lee et al. (eds.), *Vocal Fold Injection*, https://doi.org/10.1007/978-981-16-3303-4_18

of bFGF [4]. The investigators also found increased level of apoptosis at the site of bFGF injection. They suggested that the application of bFGF to acute incisional wounds accelerated apoptosis in the granulation tissue in the early phase of wound healing, and that the cell death might contribute in reduction of scarring in the late phase of healing. In a clinical study, indeed, bFGF was administered to a sutured wound on the face, trunk, and limbs by intradermal injection, and the results showed fewer incidence of hypertrophic scar formation [5].

These basic and clinical data suggest antifibrotic effects of bFGF as well as effects on stimulating wound healing mechanism.

18.1.2 Preclinical Data of bFGF on the Vocal Fold

The vocal fold scar, sulcus, and atrophy are featured with thin and/or stiff vocal fold mucosa with reduced vibratory function, which is difficult to treat. Animal and human studies have indicated excessive deposition of collagen bundles and decrease/loss of HA in the lamina propria of the vocal fold which is the main cause of vibratory dysfunction.

We have found that bFGF stimulates production of HA and suppresses production of collagen from vocal fold fibroblasts by an ELISA study [6]. The following PCR study also indicated upregulation of gene of HA synthase and MMP (collagenase) and downregulation of gene of procollagen type I [7]. These mechanisms are supposed to be effective to restore the altered histological architecture of the vocal folds. Indeed, when bFGF was locally injected into the atrophied vocal folds with age or scarred vocal folds in animal models, HA was recovered and excessive collagen disappeared or reduced [8, 9]. Vibratory function was also improved by the injection. No severe adverse events were observed. These findings suggest therapeutic potential of bFGF for the treatment of vocal fold scar and atrophy.

18.1.3 Clinical Application of bFGF Injection for Vocal Fold Scar, Sulcus, and Atrophy

Based on the preclinical data, an IRB-approved clinical trial was completed for 10 cases with vocal fold aged atrophy [10]. Ten micrograms of bFGF in 0.5 mL saline were repeatedly injected into the membranous portion (superficial lamina propria) of the vocal folds under topical anesthesia using lidocaine spray (Fig. 18.1). The results showed significant improvement of vibratory properties with improvement of voice up to 1 year. Given the positive effects, we have set up 4 serial weekly injection of bFGF for patients with vocal fold scar, sulcus, and atrophy, and reported significant improvement of voice for all pathologies in 100 cases [11]. Figure 18.2 indicates a representative case with vocal fold scar with reduced vibratory amplitude and glottic gap. Post-injection examination showed better vibration with no glottic gap.

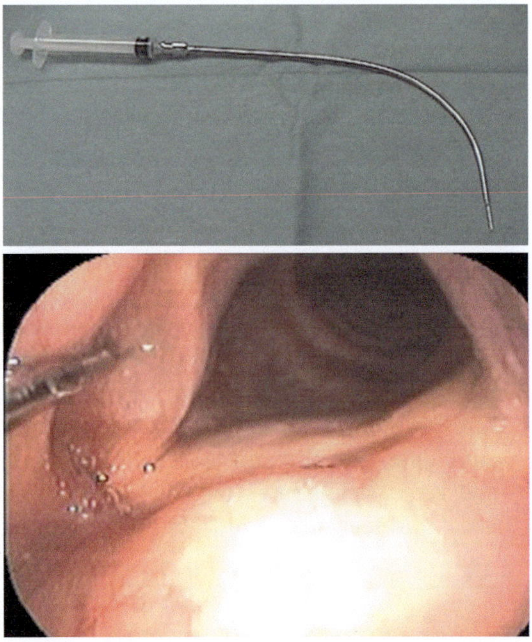

Fig. 18.1 (upper) Curved needle. (lower) intracordal injection of bFGF into the superficial layer of the lamina propria

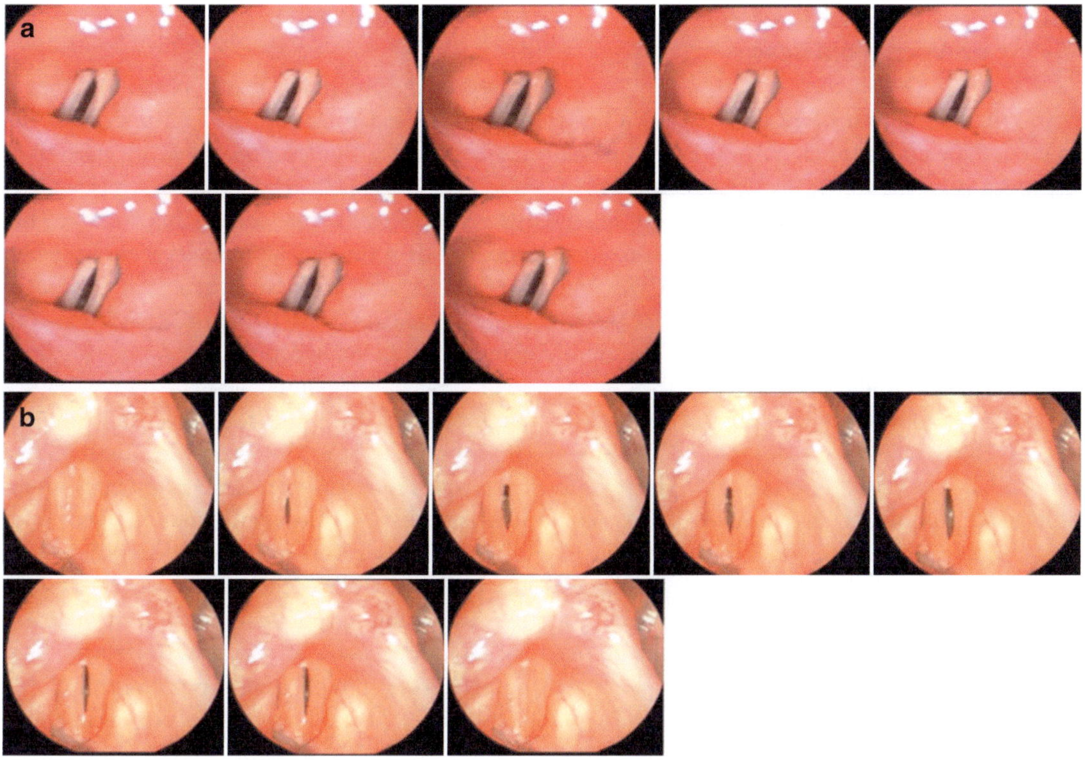

Fig. 18.2 Vocal fold scar treated with bFGF injection. (**a**) pre-injection. Little vibration was observed. (**b**) post-injection. Vibration was improved with complete glottic closure. (Cited from [11] (open access))

There have been no severe adverse events, but temporary erythema was observed in more than a half of the patients possibly because of angiogenetic effects of the growth factor. The erythema, however, were improved in 1–2 months after the injection.

The regenerative effects showed some degree of individual differences, and vocal fold atrophy showed the best results, while the effects seemed to be limited for severe scar or type II sulcus.

18.2 Hepatocyte Growth Factor

18.2.1 Anti-Fibrotic Activity

Hepatocyte growth factor (HGF) was first found as a potent mitogen for mature hepatocyte, and then several independent studies confirmed that HGF is produced by most mesenchymal cells including fibroblast in the whole body, and has multipotent activities that contribute in embryogenesis, organogenesis, angiogenesis, and tissue regeneration [12]. Given the strong angiogenesis and regenerative effects, several clinical trials have been performed or under way for patients with ischemic diseases and neural degenerative diseases.

It is also revealed that HGF has strong anti-fibrotic activity which blocks TGFb1, the key molecule of fibrosis. HGF prevents transformation of fibroblast to myofibroblast by blocking TGFb1, which leads to suppression of excessive synthase of collagen or other extracellular matrix from fibroblast. Several animal studies indicated anti-fibrotic therapeutic effects of HGF for intractable fibrotic diseases in the liver, lung, kidney, and heart.

18.2.2 Preclinical Data of HGF on Vocal Fold Scar

Given the strong anti-fibrotic activity, we have examined the effects of HGF for prevention and treatment of vocal fold scar. We first confirmed the existence of c-Met, the receptor of HGF, on the epithelium of the vocal fold [13]. In vitro study showed increased production of HA and decrease of collagen production from vocal fold fibroblasts by addition of HGF [14]. Canine studies examined therapeutic effects of local injection of solution of HGF or gelatin hydrogel of HGF on the restoration of acute or chronic scarred vocal folds [15, 16]. The results indicated significant increase of HA and decrease of collagen in the lamina propria of the vocal fold with better vibratory properties and glottic closure. HGF has proved to be effective for regeneration of the vocal fold in the cases with vocal fold scar.

18.2.3 Clinical Trial

Based on the preclinical data, a phase I/II clinical trial was performed using a GMP-compatible HGF drug for human patients with vocal fold scar and sulcus [17]. Three different doses (1, 3, 10 mg/each fold) were locally injected into the vocal folds 4 times. The patients were followed up for 6 months. The results indicated significant improvement of VHI-10 and GRBAS score at 6 months after the injections. Stroboscopic examination revealed significant increased vibratory amplitude of the vocal fold mucosa with less glottic gap. Figure 18.3 shows a representative case with moderate scar, indicating better vibratory pattern by stroboscopic examinations.

The effects had no dose-dependent differences. No severe adverse events were observed. Given the strong anti-fibrotic activity, HGF is expected to have therapeutic effects even for severe scar cases. Further clinical trials are warranted.

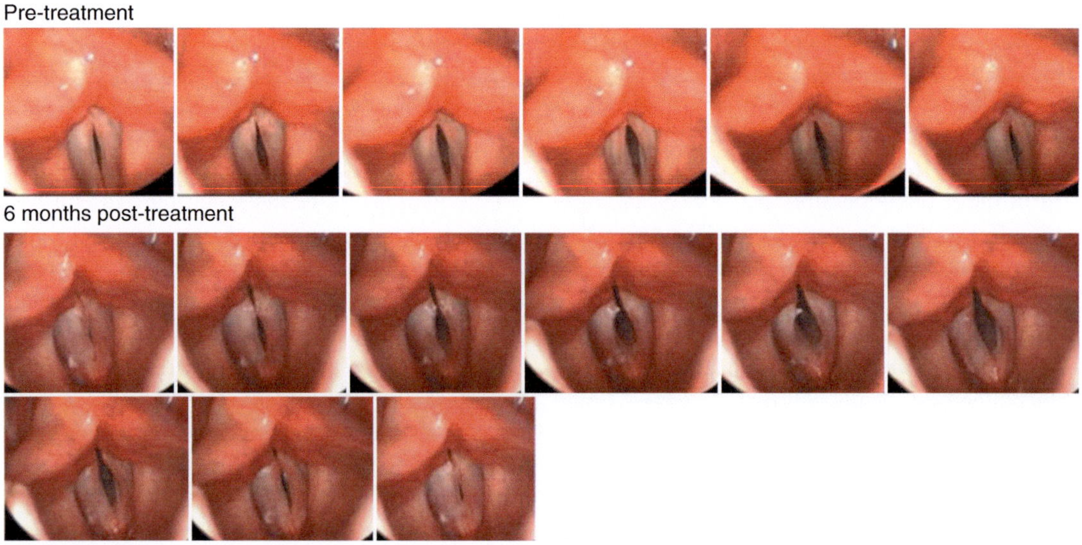

Fig. 18.3 Vocal fold scar treated with HGF injection. Pre-injection findings showed reduce vibratory amplitude with glottic gap. Post-injection findings indicated improved vibratory amplitude with glottic closure. (Cited from [16] with permission)

Key Learning Points:

- Basic fibroblast growth factor (bFGF) and hepatocyte growth factor (HGF) both have regenerative effects of the vocal fold mucosa by increasing hyaluronic acid (HA) production and resolving accumulated thick collagen bundles inside the lamina propria.
- Basic FGF and HGF are indicated for the treatment of vocal fold scar, sulcus, and atrophy.
- In general, regenerative effects occur in 1–3 months after the injection. No severe adverse events have been reported.
- There is a commercially available drug of bFGF (Fiblast®, Kaken Co., Tokyo, Japan), while there is no HGF drug approved for use for human patients.

References

1. Hong HH, Trackman PC. Cytokine regulation of gingival fibroblast lysyl oxidase, collagen, and elastin. J Periodontol. 2002;73:145–52.
2. Heldin P, Laurent TC, Heldin CH. Effect of growth factors on hyaluronan synthesis in cultured human fibroblasts. Biochem J. 1989;258:919–22.
3. Ono I, Tateshita T, Inoue M. Effects of a collagen matrix containing basic fibroblast growth factor on wound contraction. J Biomed Mater Res. 1999;48:621–30.
4. Akasaka Y, Ono I, Yamashita T, Jimbow K, Ishii T. Basic fibroblast growth factor promotes apoptosis and suppresses granulation tissue formation in acute incisional wounds. J Pathol. 2004;203(2):710–20.
5. Ono I, Akasaka Y, Kikuchi R, Sakemoto A, Kamiya T, Yamashita T, Jimbow K. Basic fibroblast growth factor reduces scar formation in acute incisional wounds. Wound Repair Regen. 2007;15(5):617–23.
6. Hirano S, Bless DM, Muñoz del Río A, Connor NP, Ford CN. Therapeutic potential of growth factors for aging voice. Laryngoscope. 2004;114:2161–7.
7. Ohno T, Jin Yoo M, Swanson ER, Hirano S, Ossoff RH, Rousseau B. Regenerative effects of basic growth factor on extracellular matrix production in aged rat vocal folds. Ann Otol Rhinol Laryngol. 2009;118:559–64.
8. Hirano S, Nagai H, Tateya I, Tateya T, Ford CN, Bless DM. Regeneration of aged vocal folds with basic fibroblast growth factor in a rat model: a preliminary report. Ann Otol Rhinol Laryngol. 2005;114:304–8.
9. Suehiro A, Hirano S, Kishimoto Y, Rousseau B, Nakamura T, Ito J. Treatment of acute vocal fold scar with local injection of basic fibroblast growth factor: a canine study. Acta Otolaryngol. 2010;130(7):844–50.
10. Hirano S, Tateya I, Kishimoto Y, Kanemaru S, Ito J. Clinical trial of regeneration of aged vocal folds with growth factor therapy. Laryngoscope. 2012;122:327–31.
11. Hirano S, Kaneko M, Kishimoto Y. Regenerative effects of local injection of basic fibroblast growth factor into the vocal fold atrophy and scarring: results of 60 cases. Ann Clin Otolaryngol. 2017;1(1):1–4.
12. Matsumoto K, Nakamura T. Hepatocyte growth factor (HGF) as a tissue organizer for organogenesis and regeneration. Biochem Biophys Res Commun. 1997;239:639–44.
13. Hirano S, Thibeault S, Bless DM, Ford CN, Kanemaru S. Hepatocyte growth factor and its receptor c-met in rat and rabbit vocal folds. Ann Otol Rhinol Laryngol. 2002;111:661–6.
14. Hirano S, Bless D, Heisey D, Ford C. Roles of hepatocyte growth factor and transforming growth factor beta1 in production of extracellular matrix by canine vocal fold fibroblasts. Laryngoscope. 2003;113:144–8.
15. Hirano S, Bless DM, Nagai H, Rousseau B, Welham NV, Montequin D, Ford CN. Growth factor therapy for vocal fold scarring in canine model. Ann Otol Rhinol Laryngol. 2004;113:777–85.
16. Kishimoto Y, Hirano S, Kitani Y, Suehiro A, Umeda H, Tateya I, Kanemaru S, Tabata Y, Ito J. Chronic vocal fold scar restoration with hepatocyte growth factor. Laryngoscope. 2010;120:108–13.
17. Hirano S, Kawamoto A, Tateya I, Mizuta M, Kishimoto Y, Hiwatashi N, Kawai Y, Tsuji T, Suzuki R, Kaneko M, Naito Y, Kagimura T, Nakamura T, Kanemaru SI. A phase I/II exploratory clinical trial for intracordal injection of recombinant hepatocyte growth factor for vocal fold scar and sulcus. J Tissue Eng Regen Med. 2018;12(4):1031–8.

19 Other Therapeutic Vocal Fold Injections

Woo-Jin Jeong

Abstract

Vocal fold (VF) injection is mainly applied for the treatment of glottic insufficiency or to manage benign VF lesions. Other therapeutic indications for VF injection that are currently available are for recurrent respiratory papillomatosis (RRP). Various other therapeutic materials for VF injections have been investigated in VF scarring, atrophy, and others. The essential principles of developing an injection material focus on substances that resemble the viscoelastic properties of the lamina propria, in turn promoting VF regeneration to restore mechanical and biochemical features of the VFs, and eventually improving the phonation and the vibratory function of the VF mucosa. Although recent approaches suggest promising therapeutic materials, most of the materials are yet limited for clinical application. Herein, we overview some of the recent studies of therapeutic materials for the VF and its clinical applications for the treatment of RRP, VF scarring, and sulcus vocalis.

Keywords

Vocal fold scar · Cidofovir · Bevacizumab Tissue engineering · Stem cell · Platelet rich plasma · Small interfering RNA Regeneration

19.1 Cidofovir and Bevacizumab

19.1.1 Clinical Application of Cidofovir or Bevacizumab on Recurrent Respiratory Papillomatosis

Recurrent respiratory papillomatosis (RRP) is a rare disease, commonly involving the larynx and the trachea, which presents with multiple papillomatous tumors. It is characterized by its unpredictable and relapsing clinical course that may potentially compromise the voice production or patency of the airway. The majority of RRP is associated with human papillomavirus (HPV) type 6 or 11. It presents with two clinical forms according to the age of onset; juvenile-onset type and adult-onset type, whereas juvenile-onset type displays a worse clinical course [1]. Surgical debulking is the primary treatment for RRP, but patients commonly undergo repeated procedures due to the relapsing nature of the disease. Thus, for those requiring more than four surgical managements per year, with rapid regrowth with airway compro-

W.-J. Jeong (✉)
Department of Otorhinolaryngology-Head & Neck Surgery, Seoul National University Bundang Hospital, Seoul National University College of Medicine, Seongnam, South Korea
e-mail: safar@snubh.org

© Springer Nature Singapore Pte Ltd. 2021
B.-J. Lee et al. (eds.), *Vocal Fold Injection*, https://doi.org/10.1007/978-981-16-3303-4_19

mise, with a distal spread of the disease, the use of adjuvant therapy is indicated [2].

Two intralesional agents are assumed as effective and applicable for adjuvant therapy. Cidofovir (Vistide®) is a cytosine nucleotide analog that could promptly incorporate into a growing DNA chain, which is perceived to inhibit the replication of herpesvirus, adenovirus, and human papillomavirus [3]. Although the Food and Drug Administration had approved its use only for Cytomegalovirus retinitis in AIDS patients, cidofovir is the most commonly used intralesional agent for RRP since 1998 [4]. There is no general protocol for injection dose and interval, but research shows that 20–40 mg in less than 4 mL is used in adults without fixed interval, rather conducted considering the clinical progression. In pediatric patients (Fig. 19.1), less than 20 mg in less than 2 mL is used with a preference of 3–6 weeks interval [5].

Bevacizumab (Avastin®) is a recombinant monoclonal antibody that prevents the growth of new vessels by binding to vascular endothelial growth factor (VEGF). Research shows that VEGF plays an important role in the growth of laryngeal papillomas [6]. In the last decade, intralesional administration of bevacizumab, with the synergistic effect of 532-nm pulsed potassium titanyl phosphate (KTP) laser photoangiolysis therapy, has demonstrated successful clinical results as adjuvant therapy for RRP [7, 8].

19.1.2 Potential Risk of Adjuvant Therapy for RRP

Although cidofovir is considered as an effective adjuvant therapy for RRP, there are controversies regarding the nephrotoxicity and malignant transformation due to cidofovir use. Concerns were derived from studies of intravenous cidofovir treated for cytomegalovirus retinitis and case reports demonstrating a carcinogenic effect after cidofovir use [9–11]. Considering these findings, the Multi-Disciplinary Task Force on RRP has provided a guideline with a recommendation of extensive patient counseling regarding the risk of treatment [12]. Several studies have attempted to investigate the potential risk of cidofovir, however, the cause of those risks remain unclear up to date. A recent long-term retrospective study suggests that clinical evidence of increased rate in dysplasia or cancer induced by intralesional injection of cidofovir is not definite [13]. As for bevacizumab, studies

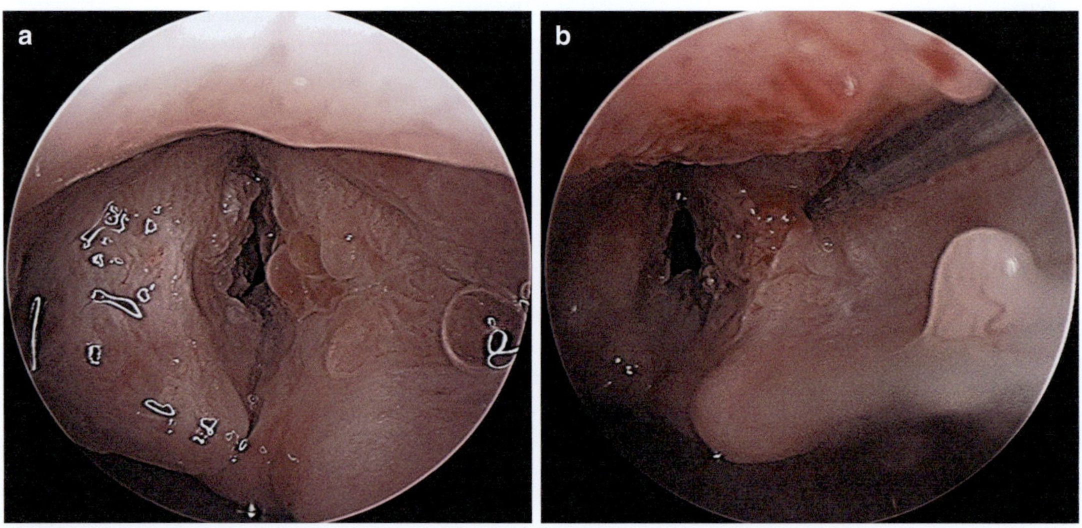

Fig. 19.1 Cidofovir injection in an 8-year-old male with recurrent respiratory papillomatosis. (**a**) Papillomatosis involving true vocal fold and false vocal fold. (**b**) Cidofovir was injected into bilateral false vocal folds. (Courtesy of Prof. Seong Keun Kwon)

regarding the possible side effects of intralesional injection of this material is currently lacking, and there have not been any considerable reports of complications up to date.

19.1.3 Outcomes of Adjuvant Therapy for RRP

Cidofovir has been widely accepted in clinical practices during the first decade of its application to RRP. However, it is difficult to evaluate the actual efficacy of the treatment, since RRP could recur from 1 week to more than 30 years after treatment [1], and only few clinical studies have provided a long-term follow-up results so far. A review of literature in 2005 provides that 40–50% of both pediatric and adult patients may achieve improved outcomes with a durable remission after cidofovir injection, and up to 20% of the patients did not respond to the therapy [12]. It is also mentioned that since the majority of the patients included were those with severe disease, the actual therapeutic outcome may have been underestimated. A recent literature review demonstrates that adult-onset RRP shows a better complete response rate (74%) to cidofovir therapy compared to Juvenile-onset RRP (56.5%) [14]. Although bevacizumab presents improving results for RRP in some clinical reports, extensive clinical studies are still required to authorize its effect. A recent systematic review of bevacizumab treated for adult-onset RRP presents that 23.3% achieved complete remission and 36.6% of the disease was controlled with continuous injections [4]. None of the reviews reported an increased rate of developing dysplasia or cancer upon administration of adjuvant therapy.

19.2 Tissue-Engineered Materials

19.2.1 Hyaluronic Acid-Based Materials

The tailored mechanical properties of injectable, bioactive, and biodegradable polymers or hydrogels offer advantages over traditional implantation materials. It has the potential to solidify materials into desired shape minimizing the invasiveness and potential trauma to patients, which also limits the risk of infection and secondary scar formation [15]. This approach has mainly involved hyaluronic acid (HA) and its derivatives due to HA's biological and biomechanical functionalities [16]. HA express high viscoelastic properties similar to the vocal fold (VF), influencing the nature of VF which is critical in phonation [17]. However, HA often degrades within 3–5 days after injecting into the VF, thus, chemical modifications of HA are required to improve the mechanical stability, and to elongate material retention [18].

The promising regenerative capacity of HA led to the development of cross-linked HA gels such as Hylan-B for the treatment of glottic insufficiency [19]. Although this divinyl sulfone cross-linked HA hydrogel strategy exhibited some improvement in a clinical trial [20], the harsh cross-linking chemistry eventually led to the loss of bioactivity, and therefore, it is currently not under clinical use. Another strategy with disulfide cross-linking chemistry using Dithiobis (propanoic dihydrazide) (DTP) was developed to form HA-DTPH macromolecules. The mild gelation reaction of HA-DTPH solution supported cell viability and proliferation in vitro, but the material was limited for clinical application due to its long gelation time forming stable hydrogels [21].

Some progress has been reported using thiols as a site of cross-linking on the HA backbone, such as Carbylan-SX and Carbylan-GSX using poly (ethylene glycol) diacrylate (PEGDA) and thiolated gelatin as a cross-linking agent, respectively. In these substances, material properties regarding degradation rates and viscoelasticity can be modulated by changing the material composition, while maintaining the biocompatibility of these gels [22, 23]. A prophylactic injection in a rabbit VF demonstrated that Carbylan-SX hydrogel can induce VF regeneration to an optimal level favoring phonation and could also minimize VF scarring after surgery [24]. Cumulative in vivo studies using Carbylan-GSX have reported pro-healing responses in rabbits and suggest administration of Carbylan-GSX in early stage of injury can improve healing and restoring vocal function [18, 25].

Injectable hydrogels with HA could also be used to deliver genetic material as a regenerative substance into the VF for active VF regeneration. A recent study assembled an injectable basic fibroblastic growth factor (bFGF) encoding plasmid DNA (pDNA) complex-loaded alginate (ALG)/HA mixture hydrogel dispersed with polycaprolactone (PCL) microspheres to enhance simultaneous regeneration of VF muscle and lamina propria (Fig. 19.2). The PCL microspheres-dispersed ALG/HA hydrogel loaded with pDNA complex was injected into a denervated rabbit VF, which demonstrated regenerative aspects of collagen composition and HA synthesis nearby the injected site. The result also exhibited a bulky agent feature of the injection leading to constant medialization of the paralyzed VF, which remained stable and effective after 24 weeks. Therefore, the pDNA (bFGF encoding) complex-loaded ALG/HA hydrogel dispersed with PCL microspheres is suggested as a candidate for injection laryngoplasty, as a bulky agent for VF augmentation which could also enhance the VF function by synthesis of collagen and HA components [26].

19.2.2 Hyaluronic Acid-Based Microgels

Biocompatible microgels provide a large surface-to-volume ratio and wide distribution of particle size to overcome the limitation of scaffolds with compromised structural integrity and mechanical stability. Hydrazide-modified HA (HAADH) and aldehyde-functionalized HA (HAALD) form microgels through inverse emulsion droplet microsphere with an average diameter of 10 μm. The microgel forms doubly cross-linked networks (DXNs) with other polymers yielding tunable viscoelasticity similar to canine VF tissues [27]. These HA-microgel presents flexible extensibility with comparable elastic shear moduli to those of VF lamina propria without adverse effect on the viability and proliferation of fibroblasts, displaying the potential of application for VF regeneration [28]. In vivo study of HA-gelatin based microgel injection into rats following VF stripping resulted in significantly lower macrophage count compared to the saline injected group at day 28, suggesting that the HA-gelatin microgels do not significantly induce inflammatory response in the VFs [29]. Due to these results, HA-based microgels are expected as an injection material for VF regeneration, but long-term in vivo study results are yet to be demonstrated.

19.2.3 Synthetic Polymer Materials

Polymer-based materials are flexible in adjusting various biochemical and mechanical features, which is applicable in VF tissue engineering [30]. Polyethylene glycol (PEG)-based hydrogel (PEG30) can be tightly controlled and modified of its mechanical properties, mesh size, degradation rate, and bioactivity. After 30 days of in vitro static culture of porcine VF fibroblasts encapsulated in four polyethylene glycol diacrylate (PEGDA) hydrogels, VF fibroblast extracellular matrix (ECM) properties were presented with a strong correlation with initial hydrogel mesh size and modulus. The sulfated glycosaminoglycan synthesis, elastin production, collagen deposition, and the induction of a myofibroblast phenotype depended on initial mesh size and initial elastic compressive moduli [31]. Further in vivo study was conducted by injecting PEG30 unilaterally into 16 normal canine VFs to investigate its effects on structural and functional parameters. As a result, all PEG30 injected VFs presented mucosal wave activity with low average phonation threshold pressures without any significant inflammation under microscopic examination. Three selected cases in this study, with the most superficial injection, were inspected under high-speed video analysis, which showed a minimal reduction in maximum vibratory amplitudes compared to the un-injected contralateral VF. The result implies that the presence of PEG30 does not negatively impact normal phonation or vibratory function compared to non-injected

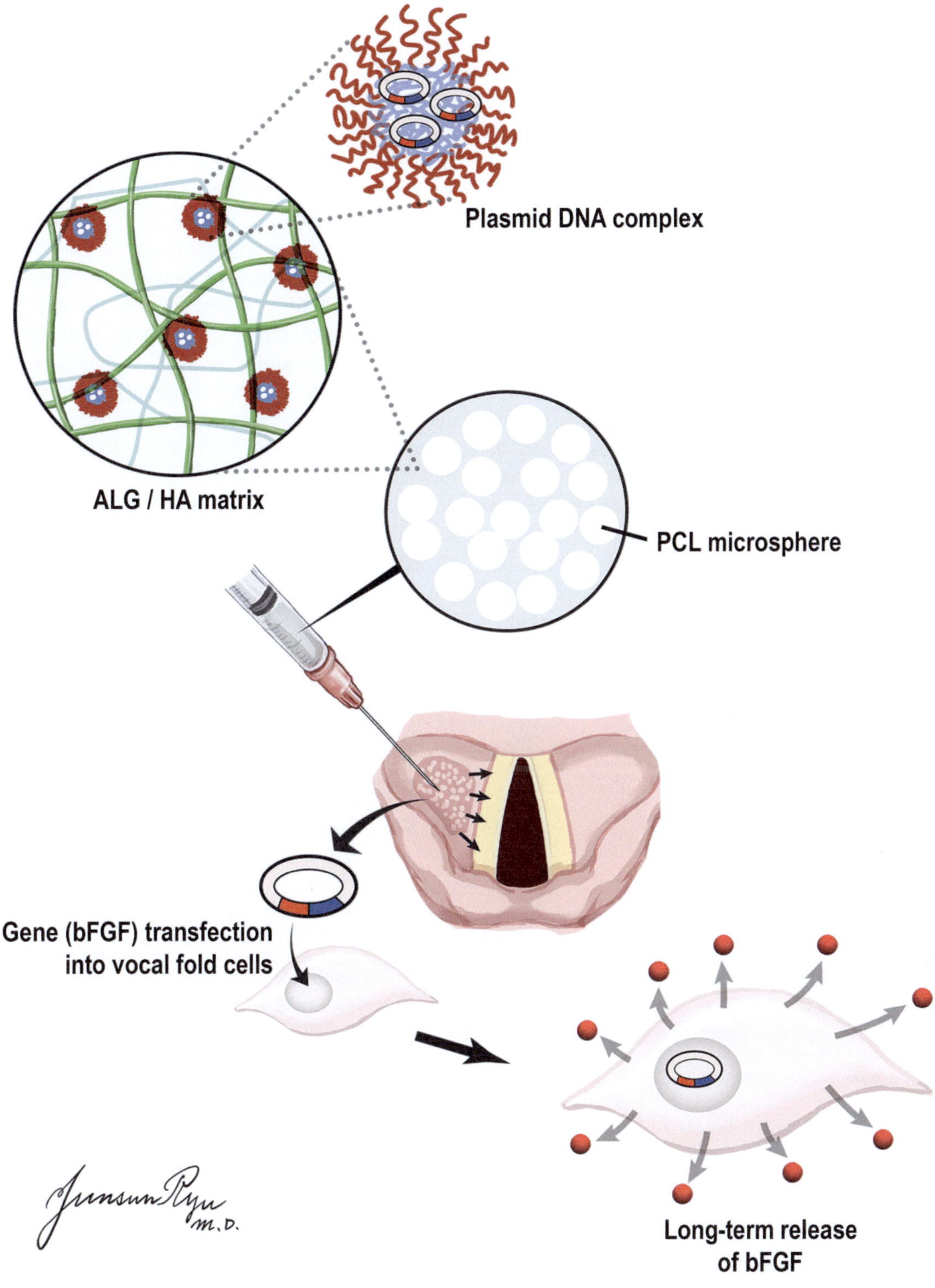

Fig. 19.2 Schematic illustrations of injectable pDNA-complex-loaded ALG/HA mixture hydrogel dispersed with polycaprolactone microspheres for the regeneration of paralyzed VF. (Redrawn based on [26] with permission)

VF. Time-dependent resorption of the PEG30 by phagocytosis was shown to induced minimal tissue reaction of fibrosis causing mucosal stiffness. The PEG30 hydrogel was therefore suggested as a promising biocompatible candidate for restoring deficient phonatory mucosa [32].

19.3 Stem Cell Therapy

19.3.1 Regeneration Therapy for the Vocal Folds

VF scarring is a replacement of fibrous tissue in the wound healing process after trauma, inflammation, iatrogenic lesion after surgery, or an adverse event after radiotherapy [33]. A fibrous scar tissue consists of a disorganized extracellular matrix (ECM), a consequence of losing the density of elastin, decreased hyaluronic acid, and fine type III collagen replaced by type I collagen [34]. Scar tissue formation in the superficial lamina propria alters the biomechanical properties of the VF, resulting in increased stiffness and reduced viscosity, which eventually leads to impaired voice quality [35].

Surgical procedures may attempt to resect the scar tissue and repair the wound. However, normal VF function may not fully be recovered since there is a potential risk of re-adhesion, and the recovery of the native ECM composition is limited with reduced viscoelasticity. Therefore, there are growing interests in applying regenerative medicine to the management of VF scarring. The intention of regenerative therapy on the VF is to fully repair the native ECM composition, in turn restoring the biomechanical properties of VF tissue, and eventually recovering the normal voice quality [36]. Regeneration therapy of VF is based on three elements; implementation of a scaffold, cell therapy, and use of bioactive factors [37]. Implementation of scaffold involves tissue-engineered materials mentioned in the previous section, and cell therapies are recently generating momentum in VF regeneration through stem cells. Although the number of researches is limited, stem cell therapy provides an ideal concept and presents encouraging

Table 19.1 Overview of indications and development status of injection materials for vocal fold regeneration

Materials	Indication	Development
Tissue-engineered materials		
Hyalin-B [19, 20]	Glottic insufficiency	Clinical trial
Carbylan-SX/GSX [24, 25]	Vocal fold scarring/ regeneration	In vivo study
Basic FGF-loaded alginate/HA hydrogel [52]	Vocal fold atrophy Glottic insufficiency	In vivo study
Hydrazide-modified HA and aldehyde-functionalized HA microgels [28, 29]	Vocal fold scarring/ regeneration	In vivo study
PEG-based hydrogel (PEG30) [31, 32]	Vocal fold scarring/ regeneration	In vivo study
Stem cell therapy		
Bone marrow-derived MSC [45]	Vocal fold scarring/ regeneration	Phase I/II clinical trial
Adipose-derived stem cells [44]	Vocal fold regeneration	In vivo study
Others		
Platelet-rich plasma [48]	Vocal fold scarring/ regeneration	In vivo study
Small interfering RNA based gene therapy [51]	Vocal fold scarring/ regeneration	In vivo study

FGF fibroblast growth factors, *HA* hyaluronic acid, *PEG* polyethylene glycol, *MSC* mesenchymal stem cell results in preclinical studies. Table 19.1 presents the overview of indications and developments of the injection materials for regeneration therapy.

19.3.2 Preclinical Study of Stem Cell Therapy

Mesenchymal stem cells (MSCs) are multipotent stromal cells most often harvested from adipose tissue or bone marrow [38]. They are easily harvested and expanded with regenerative function, therefore the therapeutic effects of MSCs on VF scarring have been investigated over the past few decades. MSCs are shown to migrate to the injured site of the VF and induce wound healing by increasing the expression of hepatocyte growth factor (HGF) [39].

Numerous in vivo studies demonstrate promising effects on wound healing and regeneration of injured VFs by local administration of MSCs into scarred VFs. In an in vivo canine study, autologous MSCs injection prior to injury presented better regeneration of VF and reduced scar tissue compared to saline controls [40]. Bone marrow-derived MSCs from a mouse were shown to promote VF wound healing in a rabbit model when it was injected immediately after mechanical injury. The treatment group in this study presented with improved morphologic features and viscoelasticity [41]. Human MSCs injected into a scarred rabbit VF also demonstrated improvement in the healing process compared to untreated scarred VFs [42, 43]. Compared to the untreated group, scarred VFs of rabbit injected with human MSCs exhibited improved dynamic viscosity and elastic modulus, also displaying reduced thickness of lamina propria and collagen type I content under histologic analysis. Adipose-derived stem cells (ASC) were also studied by injecting into an acutely injured rabbit VFs. As a result, ASC injected vocal folds exhibited significantly less inflammation with reduced hypertrophy of lamina propria and fibrosis, compared to control groups [44].

Other various types of stem cells, such as adipose-derived stem cells (ASCs), human embryogenic stem cells (hESCs), and induced pluripotent stem cells (iPSCs) are under investigation for stem cell therapy of VF regeneration. Numerous preclinical studies on various types of stem cells provide encouraging results. However, clinical trials for treating scar formations on humans are lacking. Ongoing clinical trials on VF regeneration are expected to assist in progression in this field.

19.3.3 Clinical Trial of Stem Cell for VF Regeneration

The first phase I/II clinical trial using bone marrow-derived MSCs on the treatment of VF scarring has recently been published [45]. In this study, 16 patients were treated with scar resection followed by autologous MSC injection ($0.5–2 \times 10^6$ MSCs/patients) and were monitored for 1 year. The results show that VF vibration and elasticity in 62–75% of the patients were significantly improved under digitalized analysis of high-speed laryngoscopy and phonation pressure threshold. Patients' subjective ratings using the voice handicap index scale also showed a significant improvement in half of the patients, without any reports of serious adverse events or minor side effects.

Although some concerns regarding surgical intervention and patient selection were pointed out [46], the study suggests that local injection of autologous MSCs into scarred VFs offers a safe and feasible therapeutic option. Randomized controlled and comparative studies are expected in the future to confirm the efficacy of stem cell therapy on VF regeneration.

19.4 Platelet-Rich Plasma

Platelets contain several growth factors which enable platelet-rich plasma (PRP) to express beneficial effects on wound healing with low side-effect profile. Thus, PRP is widely applicable in medical fields, especially in many surgical specialties, but PRPs were only recently introduced for VF injection. In a recent study, PRP was injected into a linear wound of VFs in 12 rabbits with normal saline injection into the contralateral side. The morphologic analysis revealed a decrease in granulation tissue compared to normal saline injected VF, but the difference in surface irregularity and atrophic change under visual inspection was not significant. Histologic analysis of PRP injected VFs demonstrated less significant inflammation and collagen deposition. Marked expression of growth factors such as PDGF, TGF-β, VEGF, and EGF was observed 14 days after surgery, whereas it was no longer significant after 12 weeks [47]. In another recent study, PRP absorbed gelfoam was applied onto a stripped lamina propria of rat VF. The result suggested that PRP accelerates epithelization of injured rat VFs by inducing EGFR secretion and may prevent scar formation [48]. Although PRP is known to benefit the healing process by promoting growth factor aggregation, more preclinical studies are required to be accepted as a promising potential material for clinical application.

19.5 Gene Therapy

Small interfering RNA (siRNA)-based therapy aims to regulate Smad3, a key biomedical signaling protein and is expected to provide a direct, localized modulation of fibrosis [49]. TGF-β is known as a regulator for development of fibrosis and wound healing which activates its growth factor pathway through the Smad family of proteins [50]. Smad3 siRNA has been shown to alter TGF-β-induced collagen mRNA expression in an in vitro study [49]. Recent in vivo study demonstrated that Smad3 expression, which is increased following VF injury, was significantly reduced in response to injection of lipitoid + siRNA injection [51]. As with the fundamental studies, further in vivo investigations are warranted for the progress of genetic modulation therapy.

Key Learning Points:

- Cidofovir and Bevacizumab are applied as adjuvant therapy for recurrent respiratory papillomatosis under specific indications, with requirement of extensive counseling regarding the risk of treatment.
- Hyaluronic acid-based hydrogels and microgels are tissue-engineered cross-linked hyaluronic acid derivatives, presenting with promising results for vocal fold regeneration in vivo.
- Polyethylene glycol-based hydrogel is a biocompatible candidate for restoring deficient phonatory mucosa, capable of controlling its mechanical properties, mesh size, degradation rate, and bioactivity.
- Mesenchymal stem cells are easily harvested and expanded with regenerative function, offering a safe and feasible therapeutic option for vocal fold scarring.
- Albeit in its early stage of development, vocal fold injection of platelet-rich plasma and gene therapy using siRNA are expected to benefit the wound healing process of the vocal fold by supporting the growth factor pathway.

Acknowledgment Gene Huh, MD, contributed to the writing of the manuscript.

References

1. Tjon Pian Gi RE, San Giorgi MR, Slagter–Menkema L, et al. Clinical course of recurrent respiratory papillomatosis: comparison between aggressiveness of human papillomavirus-6 and human papillomavirus-11. Head Neck. 2015;37(11):1625–32.
2. Derkay CS, Wiatrak B. Recurrent respiratory papillomatosis: a review. Laryngoscope. 2008;118(7):1236–47.
3. Snoeck R, Wellens W, Desloovere C, et al. Treatment of severe laryngeal papillomatosis with intralesional injections of cidofovir [(S)-1-(3-hydroxy-2-phosphonylmethoxypropyl) cytosine]. J Med Virol. 1998;54(3):219–25.

4. Drejet S, Halum S, Brigger M, Skopelja E, Parker NP. A systematic review: outcomes in adult recurrent respiratory papillomatosis treated with intralesional cidofovir or bevacizumab. Otolaryngol Head Neck Surg. 2017;156(3):435–41.
5. Derkay CS, Volsky PG, Rosen CA, et al. Current use of intralesional cidofovir for recurrent respiratory papillomatosis. Laryngoscope. 2013;123(3):705–12.
6. Vargas SO, Healy GB, Rahbar R, et al. Role of vascular endothelial growth factor–a in recurrent respiratory papillomatosis. Ann Otol Rhinol Laryngol. 2005;114(4):289–95.
7. Zeitels SM, Lopez-Guerra G, Burns JA, Lutch M, Friedman AM, Hillman RE. Microlaryngoscopic and office-based injection of bevacizumab (Avastin) to enhance 532-nm pulsed KTP laser treatment of glottal papillomatosis. Ann Otol Rhinol Laryngol. 2009;118(9):1–24.
8. Zeitels SM, Barbu AM, Landau-Zemer T, et al. Local injection of bevacizumab (Avastin) and angiolytic KTP laser treatment of recurrent respiratory papillomatosis of the vocal folds: a prospective study. Ann Otol Rhinol Laryngol. 2011;120(10):627–34.
9. Lalezari JP, Stagg RJ, Kuppermann BD, et al. Intravenous cidofovir for peripheral cytomegalovirus retinitis in patients with AIDS: a randomized, controlled trial. Ann Intern Med. 1997;126(4):257–63.
10. Lott DG, Krakovitz PR. Squamous cell carcinoma associated with intralesional injection of cidofovir for recurrent respiratory papillomatosis. Laryngoscope. 2009;119(3):567–70.
11. Bayan S, Faquin WC, Zeitels SM. Glottic carcinoma in young patients. Ann Otol Rhinol Laryngol. 2019;128(3 suppl):25–32.
12. Derkay C, Papillomas M-DTFoRR. Cidofovir for recurrent respiratory papillomatosis (RRP): a reassessment of risks. Int J Pediatr Otorhinolaryngol. 2005;69(11):1465.
13. Hoesli RC, Thatcher AL, Hogikyan ND, Kupfer RA. Evaluation of safety of Intralesional Cidofovir for adjuvant treatment of recurrent respiratory papillomatosis. JAMA Otolaryngology–Head & Neck Surgery. 2020;146(3):231–6.
14. Gazia F, Galletti B, Freni F, et al. Use of intralesional cidofovir in the recurrent respiratory papillomatosis: a review of the literature. Eur Rev Med Pharmacol Sci. 2020;24(2):956–62.
15. Li L, Stiadle JM, Lau HK, et al. Tissue engineering-based therapeutic strategies for vocal fold repair and regeneration. Biomaterials. 2016;108:91–110.
16. Gaston J, Thibeault SL. Hyaluronic acid hydrogels for vocal fold wound healing. Biomatter. 2013;3(1):e23799.
17. Chan RW, Gray SD, Titze IR. The importance of hyaluronic acid in vocal fold biomechanics. Otolaryngol Head Neck Surg. 2001;124(6):607–14.
18. Thibeault SL, Klemuk SA, Chen X, Johnson BHQ. In vivo engineering of the vocal fold ECM with injectable HA hydrogels—late effects on tissue repair and biomechanics in a rabbit model. J Voice. 2011;25(2):249–53.
19. Hallen L, Johansson C, Laurent C. Cross-linked hyaluronan (Hylan B gel): a new injectable remedy for treatment of vocal fold insufficiency-an animal study. Acta Otolaryngol. 1999;119(1):107–11.
20. Hertegård S, Hallén L, Laurent C, et al. Cross-linked hyaluronan used as augmentation substance for treatment of glottal insufficiency: safety aspects and vocal fold function. Laryngoscope. 2002;112(12):2211–9.
21. Shu XZ, Liu Y, Luo Y, Roberts MC, Prestwich GD. Disulfide cross-linked hyaluronan hydrogels. Biomacromolecules. 2002;3(6):1304–11.
22. Caton T, Thibeault SL, Klemuk S, Smith ME. Viscoelasticity of hyaluronan and nonhyaluronan based vocal fold injectables: implications for mucosal versus muscle use. Laryngoscope. 2007;117(3):516–21.
23. Kazemirad S, Heris HK, Mongeau L. Viscoelasticity of hyaluronic acid-gelatin hydrogels for vocal fold tissue engineering. J Biomed Mater Res B Appl Biomater. 2016;104(2):283–90.
24. Hansen JK, Thibeault SL, Walsh JF, Shu XZ, Prestwich GD. In vivo engineering of the vocal fold extracellular matrix with injectable hyaluronic acid hydrogels: early effects on tissue repair and biomechanics in a rabbit model. Ann Otol Rhinol Laryngol. 2005;114(9):662–70.
25. Duflo S, Thibeault SL, Li W, Shu XZ, Prestwich G. Effect of a synthetic extracellular matrix on vocal fold lamina propria gene expression in early wound healing. Tissue Eng. 2006;12(11):3201–7.
26. Kim IG, Park MR, Choi YH, et al. Regeneration of paralyzed vocal fold by the injection of plasmid DNA complex-loaded hydrogel bulking agent. ACS Biomater Sci Eng. 2019;5(3):1497–508.
27. Jia X, Yeo Y, Clifton RJ, et al. Hyaluronic acid-based microgels and microgel networks for vocal fold regeneration. Biomacromolecules. 2006;7(12):3336–44.
28. Sahiner N, Jha AK, Nguyen D, Jia X. Fabrication and characterization of cross-linkable hydrogel particles based on hyaluronic acid: potential application in vocal fold regeneration. J Biomater Sci Polym Ed. 2008;19(2):223–43.
29. Coppoolse JM, Van Kooten T, Heris HK, et al. An in vivo study of composite microgels based on hyaluronic acid and gelatin for the reconstruction of surgically injured rat vocal folds. J Speech Lang Hear Res. 2014;57(2):S658–73.
30. Rosales AM, Anseth KS. The design of reversible hydrogels to capture extracellular matrix dynamics. Nat Rev Mater. 2016;1(2):1–15.
31. Liao H, Munoz-Pinto D, Qu X, Hou Y, Grunlan MA, Hahn MS. Influence of hydrogel mechanical properties and mesh size on vocal fold fibroblast extracellular matrix production and phenotype. Acta Biomater. 2008;4(5):1161–71.
32. Karajanagi SS, Lopez-Guerra G, Park H, et al. Assessment of canine vocal fold function after injection of a new biomaterial designed to treat phona-

tory mucosal scarring. Ann Otol Rhinol Laryngol. 2011;120(3):175–84.
33. Benninger MS, Alessi D, Archer S, et al. Vocal fold scarring: current concepts and management. Otolaryngol Head Neck Surg. 1996;115(5):474–82.
34. Friedrich G, Dikkers F, Arens C, et al. Vocal fold scars: current concepts and future directions. Consensus report of the Phonosurgery Committee of the European Laryngological Society. Eur Arch Otorhinolaryngol. 2013;270(9):2491–507.
35. Hansen JK, Thibeault SL. Current understanding and review of the literature: vocal fold scarring. J Voice. 2006;20(1):110–20.
36. Fishman JM, Long J, Gugatschka M, et al. Stem cell approaches for vocal fold regeneration. Laryngoscope. 2016;126(8):1865–70.
37. Long JL. Tissue engineering for treatment of vocal fold scar. Curr Opin Otolaryngol Head Neck Surg. 2010;18(6):521–5.
38. Burt RK, Loh Y, Pearce W, et al. Clinical applications of blood-derived and marrow-derived stem cells for nonmalignant diseases. JAMA. 2008;299(8):925–36.
39. Ohno S, Hirano S. Kanemaru Si, et al. role of circulating MSCs in vocal fold wound healing. Laryngoscope. 2012;122(11):2503–10.
40. Kanemaru S-I, Kojima H, Hirano S, et al. Regeneration of the vocal fold using autologous mesenchymal stem cells. Ann Otol Rhinol Laryngol. 2003;112(11):915–20.
41. Kim Y-M, Yi T, Choi J-S, et al. Bone marrow-derived clonal mesenchymal stem cells as a source of cell therapy for promoting vocal fold wound healing. Ann Otol Rhinol Laryngol. 2013;122(2):121–30.
42. Hertegård S, Cedervall J, Svensson B, et al. Viscoelastic and histologic properties in scarred rabbit vocal folds after mesenchymal stem cell injection. Laryngoscope. 2006;116(7):1248–54.
43. Svensson B, Nagubothu RS, Cedervall J, et al. Injection of human mesenchymal stem cells improves healing of scarred vocal folds: analysis using a xenograft model. Laryngoscope. 2010;120(7):1370–5.
44. De Bonnecaze G, Chaput B, Woisard V, et al. Adipose stromal cells improve healing of vocal fold scar: morphological and functional evidences. Laryngoscope. 2016;126(8):E278–85.
45. Hertegård S, Nagubothu SR, Malmström E, LeBlanc K. Treatment of vocal fold scarring with autologous bone marrow-derived human mesenchymal stromal cells—first phase I/II human clinical study. Stem Cell Res Ther 2020;11(1):1–11.
46. Mattei A, Magalon J, Velier M, Dignat-George F, Giovanni A, Sabatier F. Commentary about mesenchymal stem cells and scarred vocal folds. Stem Cell Res Ther. 2020;11:1–2.
47. Woo SH, Jeong H-S, Kim JP, et al. Favorable vocal fold wound healing induced by platelet-rich plasma injection. Clin Exp Otorhinolaryngol. 2014;7(1):47.
48. Cobden SB, Oztürk K, Duman S, et al. Treatment of acute vocal fold injury with platelet-rich plasma. J Voice. 2016;30(6):731–5.
49. Paul BC, Rafii BY, Gandonu S, et al. Smad3: an emerging target for vocal fold fibrosis. Laryngoscope. 2014;124(10):2327–31.
50. Leask A, Abraham DJ. TGF-β signaling and the fibrotic response. FASEB J. 2004;18(7):816–27.
51. Hiwatashi N, Kraja I, Benedict PA, et al. Nanoparticle delivery of RNA-based therapeutics to alter the vocal fold tissue response to injury. Laryngoscope. 2018;128(5):E178–83.
52. Choi YH, Kim SH, Kim IG, Lee JH, Kwon SK. Injectable basic fibroblast growth factor-loaded alginate/hyaluronic acid hydrogel for rejuvenation of geriatric larynx. Acta Biomater. 2019;89:104–14.

MIX
Papier aus verantwortungsvollen Quellen
Paper from responsible sources
FSC® C105338

If you have any concerns about our products,
you can contact us on
ProductSafety@springernature.com

In case Publisher is established outside the EU,
the EU authorized representative is:
Springer Nature Customer Service Center GmbH
Europaplatz 3, 69115 Heidelberg, Germany

Printed by Libri Plureos GmbH
in Hamburg, Germany